ABC OF OBESITY

Eat Wise, Cut Back On Size

USA, This Is Why You're Fat!

A humoristic and confronting *"Old World"* view on *"New World"* eating habits.

List of nutrition values in fattening American foods and meals.

SIZE IS EVERYTHING!

By Herman de Brock Jr.

HERMAN DE BROCK JR.

ISBN: 1495344223
ISBN-13: 978-1495344220

Cover picture: "Octuple Bypass Burger"®.
Courtesy of "Heart Attack Grill"®.

Source:

FAO Food Balance Sheets 2005-2007

http://www.aicr.orghttp://chartsbin.com
Ecological association of rising incidence of esophageal adenocarcinoma with dietary carbohydrate intake - Dr. Vijay S. Khiani

http://en.wikipedia.org/wiki/List_of_countries_by_food_energy_intake
http://livinlavidalowcarb.com/blog/typical-high-carb-american-diet-leads-to-cancer-of-the-esophagus-study-finds/1310
http://publications.usa.gov/epublications/reveal-fats/reveal-fats.htm

CONTENTS

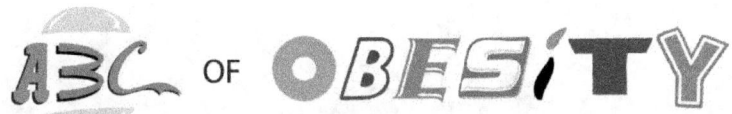

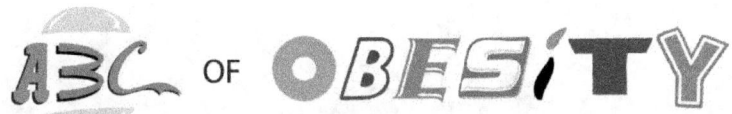

Foreword

Obesity is a life threatening worldwide epidemic, spreading rapidly throughout the (western) world. Obesity originated in the USA where corporate culture has caused portion sizes to grow completely out of proportion over the last fifty years.

The first thought that may enter an average European's mind when thinking about the USA is "Fat People". "Everything is bigger in America, especially Americans themselves!" The reason that so many Americans are overweight is not hard to figure out for Old-World folks, considering American eating habits. From spreading mayonnaise on bread to massive food portions like (chicken fried) steaks that wouldn't even fit on a humble European plate, and from deep frying vegetables to drinking enormous amounts of soft drinks.

Everything in the USA seems to have to be X-large, King-size, Super-size, Double, Triple, and Jumbo! It looks like a bunch of kids had their way with al the menus.

I'm from the Netherlands, Europe, (Holland that is) and I've had the opportunity to visit your magnificent country many times. I still find it hard to get the nutrition I'm used to and not to gain weight after a short visit.

After many visits to your great country, being a big fan of New World cooking, I felt compelled to write this book from an outsider's view, to help build awareness of the nutritional values of foods in America.

There is a major difference in food consumption between Europe and the USA though we generally use the same products. "Everything is the same but it's different!"

The ABC of obesity is meant as a kitchen table nutritional reference book with a humoristic view of American eating habits through the eyes of one Dutch man (hopefully showing that not everything in The Netherlands is as crazy as you all might think

The A B C of why you are FAT !

The truth is one can do without most, if not all of the following items, really!! If for some kind of strange reason you feel that you need to use one or more of these food items, do use them VERY MODERATELY!!

A. All You Can Eat...

B. Bacon & Eggs, Biscuits & Gravy, Burgers & Beer, Burritos, Blackened Meat (Not fattening but very unhealthy)

C. Cake, Candybars, Cereals, Cheese, Chicken/Country Fried, Chocolate, Cola, Corndogs, Cream

D. Deep Fried, Diet-Soda, Doggy Bags, Donuts, Dressing

E. Eating Contests, Energy Drinks & Energizers, Extra...

F. Fast Food, Footlong... Free Refills, Fried, Fries, Fruit Drinks

G. Giant... Gravy, Grilled

H. Hamburgers, Hot Dogs

I. Ice-Cream, Inbetweens

J. Jell-o, Jelly, Jumbo... Junk Food

K. King-size... Kentucky-Fried-Chicken, Ketchup

L. Light, Low-Fat, Low-Sugar

M. Macaroni & Cheese, Mayonnaise, McDonalds, Milkshakes

N. Nachos, Nonfat (yeah, right)

O. Obesity, Over-consumption, Overeating, Oversized

P. Pancakes, Pies, Pizza, Potato-chips

Q. Quarter Pounder, Quesadillas

R. Ribs

S. Sugar, Salt, Sandwiches, Sauce, Sausages, Smoothies, Snacks, Soda-pop, Steak, Super-size... Syrup

T. Take-out, TV Dinners

U. Ultra-Thin Slices (and lots of them), USA vs. EUROPE

V. Vanilla

W. Waffles, Whipped Cream

X. XXL

Y. Yams, Yoghurt-Drinks, You

Z. Zero-sugar

RDI - GDA

All the nutrient values described in this book are based on the Reference Daily Intake or Recommended Daily Intake (R.D.I.) for the an average women's 2000 calorie diet according to the US Food and Drug Administration (FDA) and the European version, the Guideline Daily Amount (G.D.A.). The values represent the RDI Based on an average women's and children's 2000 calorie diet. For a man it should be 2500-2700 calories so the values will be 25%-35% higher.

Remember that these are average guidelines and can vary from one person to the next.

RDI is the daily intake level of a nutrient that is considered to be sufficient to meet the requirements of 97-98% of healthy individuals in every demographic in the United States. The FDA (Food and Drug Administration) uses Daily Values (DVs) for food labeling, these values are printed on nutrition facts labels. DVs for the following macronutrients are Daily Reference Values (DRVs). The DV's used by the FDA for vitamins and minerals are the Reference Daily Intake (or Recommended Daily Intake) (RDI's) listed here. For people 4 years or older, eating 2,000 calories per day, the RDIs are:

The GDA is the European equivalent of the RDI. Guideline Daily Amounts or GDAs are a guide to how many calories and nutrients people can consume each day for a healthy, balanced diet. The GDA values shown on a food or drink label should be those for an average "adult's" daily consumption. Food Drink Europe (F.D.E.), the former CIAA (Confederation of the food and drink industries of the EU (Confédération des industries agro-alimentaires de l'UE)) established these GDA values for "adults"

Sodium is a part of salt and can be converted to salt content by multiplying it by 2.5.

Recommended Daily Intake (R.D.I.) According to the F.D.A. (USA)			Guideline Daily Amount (G.D.A.) According to the C.I.A.A. (EU)		
	Women	Men		Women	Men
Energy	2000 Calories	2500 Calories	Energy	2000 Calories	2500 Calories
Carbohydrates	300 g	375 g	Carbohydrates	270 g	340 g
Sugars	?	?	Sugars	90 g	110 g
Total Fat	65 g	80 g	Total Fat	70 g	80 g
Saturated Fat	20 g	30 g	Saturated Fat	20 g	30 g
Protein	50 g	60 g	Protein	50 g	60 g
Fiber	25 g	25 g	Fiber	25 g	25 g
Cholesterol	300 mg	?	Cholesterol	?	?
Sodium	2.4 g	2-4 g	Sodium	2.4 g	2-4 g
Salt	6 g	6 g	Salt	6 g	6 g
Potassium	4700 mg	?	Potassium	?	?

Note that the US - RDI recommends 30 g more carbs with a 2000 cal diet than the EU - GDA does, but 5 g less fat.

Source:
Eurodiet Reports and Proceedings, Public Health Nutrition, Volume 4 Number 2(A) April 2001
http://www.fooddrinkeurope.eu/
http://gda.ciaa.eu/ http://gdafacts.eu/
http://www.fda.gov/Food
http://fnic.nal.usda.gov/
www.who.int/dietphysicalactivity/publications/facts/obesity/en/
http://www.ciaa.be/documents/press_releases/CIAA_Nut_recommendation.pdf
http://en.wikipedia.org/wiki/Reference_Daily_Intake
http://en.wikipedia.org/wiki/Fda

Food Facts

* The average American needs 2,200 calories per day. Yet, the average American consumed 3,800 calories per day in 2003-2005.
Source: http://www.fao.org/economic/the-statistics-division-ess/publications-studies/statistical-yearbook/fao-statistical-yearbook-2009/d-consumption/en/

* Consuming 500 extra calories per day will cause you to gain one pound per week!
Source: http://www.bmi-calculator.net/bmr-calculator/harris-benedict-equation/calorie-intake-to-gain-weight.php

* One-third of American diet is junk food and soft drinks. Americans get about one-third of their total calories from restaurants .
Source: http://www.naturalnews.com/001109.html

* 64 percent of Americans now considered either overweight or obese. This is an immense national health problem folks!

* 58.1 percent of Americans engage in little or no physical activity.
Source: http://www.faqs.org/nutrition/Diab-Em/Dietary-Trends-American.html

* Each American eats out, on average, about 209 times per year. This includes dining in restaurants and getting take-out.
Source: http://www.wisegeek.com/how-do-steaks-served-in-restaurants-compare-with-recommended-portion-sizes.htm

* Fatty foods may cause cocaine-like addiction.
Source: http://www.cnn.com/2010/HEALTH/03/28/fatty.foods.brain/index.html?hpt=C2

* About 247 lb (112 kg) of meat is eaten per American per year. (The world's highest rate.) Beef 87.7 lbs (39.8 kg), pork 64.6 lbs (29.3 kg), poultry 92.8 lbs (42.1kg), and other meats 2 lbs (1 kg).
Source:www.ajcn.org/cgi/content/full/78/3/660S#T1
http://www.fas.usda.gov/dlp/circular/2010/livestock_poultryfull101510.pdf

* About 187 lb (85 kg) of meat is eaten per Dutchman per year. (Germans eat even less: 130 lbs (59 kg).) Beef 43 lbs (19 kg), pork 90 lbs (41 kg), poultry 50 lbs (23 kg), and other meats 5 lbs (2 kg).
Source: statline.cbs.nl/StatWeb/publication/?DM=SLNL&PA=37154&D1=0-20,22-27,42-54&D2=81,86,91,96,101-109&VW=T

* The average American eats 63 donuts per year, the average Dutch guy about 2 a year.
Source: Baltimore Sun

* The average American consumes around 160 pounds of sugar each year.
Source: http://uk.askmen.com/sports/foodcourt_150/153b_eating_well.html

* A typical restaurant serving of pasta, for example, is 10 times a recommended single portion size!
Source: http://www.thatsfit.com/2009/05/29/out-of-control-portion-sizes/

* According to the National Soft Drink Association (NSDA), consumption of soft drinks is now over 600 12-ounce servings per person per year (a 10-fold since 1942). That's 56 gallons (212 ltr). In Holland it's 25 gallons (95.8 ltr) per person per year.

* The USA is the world's second leading ice-cream consumer with 5.7 gallons (21.6 liter) per person per year. For comparison: The Dutch and the English consume about 2.1 gallons (8 liter) pp per year.

* Unsaturated fat molecules contain less energy (calories) than saturated fat.

Examples of foods containing a high proportion of saturated fat include dairy products (especially cream and cheese but also butter and ghee); animal fats such as suet, tallow, lard and fatty meat; coconut oil, cottonseed oil, palm kernel oil, chocolate, and some prepared foods.

Foods containing unsaturated fats include avocado, nuts, and vegetable oils such as canola, and olive oils. Meat products contain both saturated and unsaturated fats.

Olive oil and Canola oil contain the highest percentage of unsaturated fats and are therefore highly recommended for cooking.

Although unsaturated fats are healthier than saturated fats, the Food and Drug Administration (FDA) recommendation stated that the amount of unsaturated fat consumed should not exceed 30% of one's daily caloric intake (or 67 grams given a 2000 Calorie diet).
Source: http://www.businessweek.com/lifestyle/content/healthday/635088.html

* Waffle House ® and Cracker Barrel® will not publish nutritional data on their food!
Source: http://www.wafflehouse.com/contact-us/faqs/3-does-waffle-house-publish-nutritional-information
http://www.crackerbarrel.com/about-us/company-faqs/

* Obesity has reached epidemic proportions globally, with more than 1 billion adults overweight - at least 300 million of them clinically obese. According to the World Health Organisation.

* Obesity and overweight pose a major risk for chronic diseases, including type 2 diabetes, cardiovascular disease, hypertension and stroke, and certain forms of cancer. The key causes are increased consumption of energy-dense foods high in saturated fats and sugars, and reduced physical activity.

* Only 3% of U.S. citizens adhere to the 4 key healthy lifestyle characteristics: not smoking, maintaining healthy weight, eating adequate amounts of fruits and vegetables, and exercising regularly.
Source: http://www.annals.org/content/144/8/621.full.pdf

* Food portions weren't always so massive. Back in the 1950s, McDonald's offered just one size of French fries; that size, containing 210 calories, is now the smallest on the menu -- the largest contains a belt-busting 610 calories. The 7-Eleven Double Gulp, a 64-ounce soda (nearly 800 calories) is 10 times the size of a Coca-Cola when it was first introduced in 1886. In fact, beverage sizes have ballooned so much over the past generations, auto manufacturers have had to install larger cup holders to accommodate them.

Source:
http://www.thatsfit.com/2009/05/29/out-of-control-portion-sizes/

Food Quotes

"Listen to your body, not your culture."
Joseph SB Morse, The Evolution Diet

"More die in the United States of too much food than of too little."
John Kenneth Galbraith

"Americans have more food to eat than any other people and more diets to keep them from eating it"
Unknown

"If we're not willing to settle for junk living, we certainly shouldn't settle for junk food."
Sally Edwards

"Cheating on weekends means you're willing to be 5/7ths healthy."
Jim Mullanaphy

"Leave the drugs in the chemist's pot if you can heal the patient with food."
Hippocrates

"Ask your child what he wants for dinner only if he's buying."
Fran Lebowitz

"Once you're sensitized to the negative effects of unhealthy choices, it gets easier to turn down what used to seem impossible to resist." *Mark Sisson, The Primal Blueprint*

"You are what you eat - and perhaps surprisingly, you also are what your ancestors ate."
Jack Challem

"There is simply no moral, ethical or social justification for marketing junk food to children."
Susan Linn, Consuming Kids: The Hostile Takeover of Childhood.

"...we allowed the nutrition experts and the advertisers to shake our confidence in common sense, tradition, the testimony of our senses, and the wisdom or our mothers and grandmothers."
Michael Pollan, In Defense of Food.

"The commonest form of malnutrition in the western world is obesity."
Mervyn Deitel.

"I like rice. Rice is great if you're hungry and want 2000 of something."
Mitch Hedberg.

"Americans can eat garbage, provided you sprinkle it liberally with ketchup, mustard, chili sauce, Tabasco, cayenne pepper or any other condiment that destroys the original flavor of the dish."
Henry Miller.

"Americans eat food, fully aware that small amounts of poison have been added to improve its appearance and delay putrefaction."
John Cage

"Water is the most neglected nutrient in your diet but one of the most vital."
Kelly Barton

"We think fast food is equivalent to pornography, nutritionally speaking."
Steve Elbert

"It's truly remarkable how successful Madison Avenue has been at indoctrinating eating habits that produce huge profits for giant multinational corporations - and developing devastating health consequences for consumers - into generations of society."
Mark Sisson, The Primal Blueprint

"We are living in a world today where lemonade is made from artificial flavors and furniture polish is made from real lemons."
Mad Magazine

"If you're going to America, bring your own food."
Fran Lebowitz

"Preach not to others what they should eat, but eat as becomes you, and be silent."
Epictetus

"As for butter versus margarine, I trust cows more than chemists."
Joan Gussow

"It's bizarre that the produce manager is more important to my children's health than the pediatrician."
Meryl Streep

"In general, mankind, since the improvement in cookery, eats twice as much as nature requires."
Benjamin Franklin

Source:

http://foodquotes.net
http://thinkexist.com/quotations/food/3.html
http://cavemanforum.com/index.php?topic=2255.5;wap2

A.

All You Can Eat...

Now this is just asking for it. An invitation to come in and overeat until you're completely stuffed! And you've got to get your money's worth of course, how can you resist? What person in his right mind can truly believe that an all you can eat for $ 5.99 meal could be healthy for you, or even worth eating. No really. Think about it! A restaurant has to make money. They use a lot of (cheap) fat, sugars and batter in preparing these buffets, these will help you feel full very fast. Cheap food means low-nutrition, high-calorie junk food!

Overindulging will force your stomach to expand, so next time you will be hungrier faster and able to eat even more.

B.

Bacon & Eggs

"Ye olde" English style breakfast (or part of it). This dates back from the days where folks would do physically hard work for 12 to 16 hours a day. Yes, your body would need a big breakfast like that back then. It doesn't really nowadays; most of the hard labor at the present is being done with machines, with maybe some exceptions.

On average, two eggs and three strips of bacon will clog you with 350 calories, 28 gr. Fat - 43% RDI*, 10 gr. Saturated Fat - 50% RDI, 460mg Cholesterol - 138% RDI!

Out on the Chisholm Trail, herding cattle, I'm sure someone would need bacon & eggs for breakfast, maybe even some beans too... Nowadays, waking up with two or three slices of bread with one, maybe two slices of ham, turkey or cheese is sufficient.

See also Breakfast.

(*RDI Recommended Daily Intake based on a 2000 calorie diet according to the FDA)

Source:
http://caloriecount.about.com

Biscuits & Gravy

A little cupcake size piece of bread that seems to weigh as much as half a loaf (at least on my stomach). And eaten with some warm creamy sauce called gravy. I doubt there is anyone in Holland who has even heard of this food, let alone know where to fit it in a daily diet. See also the Gravy chapter.

Here's a little list based on 1 serving of Biscuits & Gravy:

Product	Calories	Fat	Saturated Fat	Sodium	Carbohydrates
Burger King®	410	22.0 g	6.0 g	1240 mg	43.0 g
RDI	20.5%	34%	30%	52%	14%
Chick-fil-A®	330	15.0 g	4.0 g	950 mg	43.0 g
RDI	16.5%	23%	20%	40%	14%
Shoney's®	683	31.6 g	5.0 g	2113 mg	87.7 g
RDI	34%	49%	25%	88%	29%
Whataburger®	530	36.0 g	14 g	1823 mg	52.0 g
RDI	26.5%	55%	77%	76%	17%

Source:

http://caloriecount.about.com http://www.chick-fil-a.com/?#nutritiondata
http://www.bk.com/cms/en/us/cms_out/digital_assets/files/menu_nutrition/Nation
alNutritionals.pdf
http://www.whataburger.com/browse_nutritional_info.php

Bread

See Sandwich.

Breakfast

Definitely the most important and most "skipped" meal of the day.

A regular breakfast for me would be 2 or 3 slices of bread, spread thinly with butter, and with one slice of cheese or ham/turkey or some jam each, and a glass of milk. Sometimes served with a boiled egg. This "light bread meal" is more or less a standard in The Netherlands.

The All American Breakfast: Toast, jam, eggs, cheese, sausage, bacon, beans, hash browns, coffee and fruit juice. Or this one: a stack of pancakes/waffles with syrup/cream/butter/sugar, bacon and eggs. Even Better: a whole steak with omelet, hash browns, bread and butter. For breakfast!?

Can anyone effectively eat this stuff for breakfast? Arnold Schwarzenegger maybe...

These kind of breakfasts date back from a time where people had to do hard physical work for 12 to 16 hours a day, or even longer. Sitting behind your computer screen all day calls for a somewhat lighter meal.

A couple of high-calorie examples: (Note the fat and cholesterol percentages!)

Denny's® All American Slam Two scrambled eggs with cheese, two sausage links, two bacon slices, two toast slices and hash browns.

Calories	Fat	Saturated Fat	Carbs	Cholesterol	Protein	Sodium
830	69 g (106%)	26 g (130%)	5 g (2%)	780 mg (260%)	43 g (84%)	1250 mg (63%)

IHOP® Breakfast: Omelette Feast, The Big Steak Omelette, No Pancakes. Tender strips of steak, hash browns, green peppers, onions, mushrooms, tomatoes, and cheddar cheese. Served with salsa.

Calories	Fat	Saturated Fat	Carbs	Cholesterol	Protein	Sodium
915	72 g (111%)	27 g (135%)	14 g (5%)	863 mg (287%)	53 g (104%)	690 mg (29%)

Ruby's® Breakfast Burrito

Calories	Fat	Saturated Fat	Carbs	Cholesterol	Protein	Sodium
1439	70 g (108%)	32 g (160%)	146 g (49%)	607 mg (202%)	52 g (104%)	2311 mg (96%)

Percentages R.D.I. according to the F.D.A. based on a 2000 calorie diet.

Also see the Pancakes and Waffles chapters.

Source:
http://www.livestrong.com/thedailyplate
http://caloriecount.about.com/calories-rubys-diner-breakfast-burrito-i690035
http://www.dennys.com/LiveImages/enProductImage_790.pdf

15

Burgers & Beer

What's more American than a hamburger? Americans eat 2 burgers a week on average. Sugared bread, grilled ground beef, mustard, mayo, ketchup... A calorie-bomb!

A Regular, Single Patty Hamburger contains from 250 calories up and a regular bottle of beer (12 fl oz / 0.35 ltr) about 150 calories (103 cal For a light-beer). That's 400 calories! For a woman that would be about 20%, and for a man 16% of your GDA (Guideline Daily Amounts) according to European standards.

A Quarter Pounder® by itself goes up to 505 calories, 25% of a woman's GDA, a Whataburger® 620 cal, a Whopper® 670 cal, a Big Tasty® with bacon 870 calories, a Triple Whopper® 1250 cal and a Western Burger® 1300 calories!! (now seriously, who really needs this?) I have seen bigger burgers in Texas and ...

The most caloric burger is the Octuple Bypass Burger® made proudly by the Heart Attack Grill® in Las Vegas. People over 350 lbs (160 kg) can eat for free there!?! Served with 8 half-pound beef patties (1800 g), 16 slices of cheese and covered in lard. The 40 slices of bacon are optional. The Quadruple Bypass Burger® was called the highest calorie burger according by the Guinness Book Of Records with 9,982 calories so the octuple must be around 18,000 calories. 32 ounces (230 to 910 g) 3.24 pounds

I do love a nice burger but I eat them very rarely compared to US standards.

Source:
http://caloriecount.about.com
http://nutrition.mcdonalds.com/nutritionexchange/nutritionfacts.pdf
http://www.whataburger.com/browse_nutritional_info.php
http://www.bk.com/cms/en/us/cms_out/digital_assets/files/menu_nutrition/Nation
alNutritionals.pdf http://www.dennys.com/LiveImages/enProductImage_690.pdf
http://www.heartattackgrill.com en.wikipedia.org/wiki/Heart_Attack_Grill

Burritos

World famous Mexican junk food, and cheap! A single bean burrito on average contains 370 calories (chicken 390 and beef 420 cal), over 50% of your daily salt (sodium) needs, 10 grams of fat (15% RDI), and 55 grams of carbohydrates (18 % RDI). But it can be bigger and fatter of course. A cheesy potato burrito goes for 530 cal, and the grilled stuft beef burrito can instantly "stuff" you with 700 calories. Topped with the 1439 cal Ruby's® breakfast burrito.

Also see the Breakfast chapter.

Source:http://caloriecount.about.com http://www.tacobell.com/nutrition/information

Blackened Meat

As mentioned before, this meat is not very fattening by itself but extremely unhealthy, I felt I needed to reiterate it anyway. The first time I ever attended a BBQ in the Sates, I was shocked by the looks of the hot dog sausages, completely black. When asked if they weren't burned but I was told that they were nice and crispy this way, and the burned taste would be subdued by the ketchup and what not. The black stuff was only "charcoal" and therefore "harmless". That didn't add up I thought.

I read a Cajun cooking book not much later and there was a chapter on "blackened meat". Burn the meat in the flame?! *"Crematory meat"* is what some cooks in Holland call it.

People who regularly eat very well-done red meat that is burned or charred may increase their risk of pancreatic cancer by almost 60 percent, according to a study by the University of Minnesota in 2009.

Source:
http://www.med.umn.edu/news/pancreaticcancer042209/home.html

C.

Cake

Happy Birthday! On average a slice of birthday cake carries around 300 calories.

Candy Bars

I have counted 92 different candy bars sold in the USA! That must be a dream for any kid because you need to try them all before you can choose right? The British have over 60 and in Holland, there are just over 20 different kinds available.

A Mars® Bar* in The Netherlands (51 g) contains: 230 calories, sugar - 32 g (36% GDA**), fat - 9 g (13% GDA), Saturated Fat - 5 g (26% GDA).
The Milky Way® Bar* in the USA (58.12 g) contains: 260 calories, sugar - 35 g (39% GDA), fat - 10 g (15% GDA), Saturated Fat - 7 g (35% GDA).

* The non-US Mars® Bar is similar to the The Milky Ways® Bar sold in the USA. ** GDA according to the CIAA.

Source: http://www.chocoladeinbalans.nl/ http://www.milkywaybar.com
http://www.ciaa.be/documents/press_releases/CIAA_Nut_recommendation.pdf
http://en.wikipedia.org/wiki/List_of_chocolate_bar_brands

Carbohydrates

See Sugar.

Cereals

Except for regular cornflakes but the cereals sold in the States seem to be just completely from another world. They come in all colors of the rainbow (do people really eat this?), looking more like dried dog-food to me than anything else, chocolate covered candy-puffs which should probably be regarded as a treat rather then breakfast, and edible cartoon-characters to make eating more "fun". That's probably why some people like to eat bowls of them, sometimes with added sugar and even whipped cream!

Most cereals are a reasonable addition to your breakfast, however: The advised serving size is around one cup (30 g), this is not even half a bowl, let alone more than one full bowl!

Here's a list of some of America's favorite cereals with RDIs based on a 2000 calories diet. *(Note the serving sizes)* Servings are without milk or added sugars.

Product	Serving Size	Calories	Fat	Sodium	Carbs.	Sugar
Corn Flakes	1 cup (28.0 g)	101	0.2 g	202 mg	24.4 g	2.9 g
RDI		5%	0%	8%	8%	
Cocoa Puffs®	3/4 cup (27.0 g)	110	1.5 g	150 mg	23.0 g	12.0 g
RDI		6%	2%	6%	8%	
Cheerios®	1 cup (30.0 g)	110	2.0 g	210 mg	22.0 g	1.0 g
RDI		6%	3%	8.8%	7%	
Froot Loops®	1 cup (30.0 g)	118	0.6 g	141 mg	26.7 g	12.5 g
RDI		6%	1%	6%	9%	
Frosted Flakes®	3/4 cup (31.0 g)	114	0.1 g	143 mg	28.2 g	12.0 g
RDI		6%	0%	6%	9%	
Honey Nut Cheerios®	3/4 cup (28.0 g)	110	2.0 g	210 mg	22.0 g	9.0 g
RDI		6%	3%	9%	7%	
Lucky Charms®	3/4 cup (27.0 g)	110	1.0 g	190 mg	22.0 g	12.0 g
RDI		6%	2%	8%	7%	
Rice Krispies®	1 1/4 cup (33.0 g)	128	0.3 g	229 mg	28.1 g	3.1 g
RDI		6%	0%	10%	9%	
Wheaties®	1 cup (30.0 g)	110	1.0 g	210 mg	24.2 g	4.0 g
RDI		6%	2%	9%	8%	

Source:
http://caloriecount.about.com

Cheese

Cheese on burgers, hot dogs, eggs, fries, pizza, tacos, chicken, chips, cookies, wraps, sandwiches, salads, chili, macaroni, in jars, sprinklers, boxes, spray cans, tons of cheese! There is hardly any food left where someone hasn't figured out a way to add cheese to it. We all know that cheese is fat; around 25%, except maybe for cottage cheese, which is also fairly low in calories. Yet we seem to crave cheese like maniacs. 30 pounds (13.6 kg) of cheese, and growing, is consumed per person per year in the US; that's 2.5 lbs per month. The French (of course) are world leaders with 53.7 lbs (24.4 kg).

Kraft® seems to be the largest manufacturer of "Pasteurized prepared (processed) cheese products". This designation, which appears particularly on many American store- and generic-branded singles, actually means that it doesn't meet the moisture and/or milk fat standards to be called cheese. Easy Cheese® and Velveeta® are well-known examples.

One Kraft® American Single (19 g) contains 60 cal, 4.5 g fat, 2.5 g sat. fat, 1 g carbs, 3 g protein.

Source:

http://caloriecount.about.com http://www.livestrong.com http://en.wikipedia.org/wiki/Processed_cheese

Chicken / Country Fried

I'm referring here to all food dipped in batter and deep-fried. Steak, chicken, fish, onion rings, okra, and what not. Now, we all kinda know that this cannot be the healthiest way of cooking anything. The batter will soak up fat until it's saturated. Sure it tastes nice, but why would you wanna add a layer of fat to all foods when you can grill them just as easy and get a perfect flavor?

Chocolate

Y'all ladies favorite since 1100 BC! Xocolãtl, contains the "love-drug" phenylethylamine - the same chemical that is released in your brain when you fall in love. That might be the reason it's a favorite ingredient for so many different foods. A regular Hershey bar 1.55 oz. (43 g) contains 210 cal (10.5 % GDA), 13 grams of fat (20% RDI) and 26 grams of carbs (9% RDI). Chocolate milk has about 208 cal per cup, 8.5 g of fat and almost 26 g of carbs. Not to mention the 30 mg. of cholesterol (10% RDI). A piece of chocolate cake (1/8 of 18 oz) has 235 cal, 10.5 g of fat and 34.9 g of carbs. One chocolate chip cookie sees about 78 cal, 4.5 g of fat and 9 g of carbs.

Source: http://caloriecount.about.com http://en.wikipedia.org/wiki/Chocolate

Coffee

There are no calories in a cup of coffee as long as you will not put anything in it. But of course, some milk, sugar, mocha, chocolate, caramel, whipped cream and your "missing" calories are there! A "small" 8 oz (0.24 ltr) Starbucks® Cappuccino with 2% milk is good for 80 calories, a Café Latte (just latte will get you a glass of milk in Italy) 100 calories, Mocha 130 cal and White Chocolate Mocha 200 cal. "Non-fat" milk deducts a mere 20 or 30 calories per cup while Whole Milk adds just that. And yes, the calories will double with a Grande 16 oz cup naturally!

Leading up to a fantastic Whole Milk Venti Iced 24 oz (0.7 ltr) Iced Peppermint White Chocolate Mocha with an uncanny 610 calories! Topped by the 720 calories floating in your White Chocolate CrÃ¨me Frappuccino® Blended Beverage with whipped cream. For real?

On average a European cup of coffee is about 125-150 ml (4.2-5 fl oz), 8 oz is a large cup, 16 oz is humongous to us, let alone 20 oz or even 24 oz! The amount of caffeine would drive me nuts.

Source:
http://en.wikipedia.org/wiki/Latte
http://www.starbucks.com/menu/catalog/nutrition?drink=all

Cola

A single bottle serving of Coca-Cola® has increased from 6 1/2 to 20 ounces since the 1950's. (Not even mentioning the free or cheap refills nowadays). Coca-Cola® did once contain an estimated nine milligrams of cocaine per glass, but in 1903 it was removed. Coca-Cola® still contains coca flavoring.

During the Great Depression, Pepsi® gained popularity following the introduction in 1936 of a 12-ounce bottle. "Twice as much for a nickel", referring to the Coca-Cola® standard of six ounces per bottle for the price of five cents (a nickel), instead of the 12 ounces Pepsi® sold at the same price. Regrettably introducing the "larger size competition" in the soft-drink business and the whole **"Bigger is Better"** idea.

A 12 ounce serving of Coke® or Pepsi® nowadays contains your USDA recommended daily percentage of added sugar (40g -1.41 oz) and 140 cal.

See also Soda-pop.

Source:

http://en.wikipedia.org/wiki/Coca-Cola http://en.wikipedia.org/wiki/Pepsi http://www.thatsfit.com/2009/05/29/out-of-control-portion-sizes/

Corn Dog

A kid's corn dog, 74 grams per serving contains no less than 210 calories (over 10% GDA). Fat - 11 g (17% RDI) . Carb. - 23 g (8% RDI) Sodium 530 mg (20% RDI). Might be my European mind but it doesn't sound like a healthy children's snack.

Source:

http://www.sonicdrivein.com/pdfs/menu/SonicNutritionGuide.pdf

Cream

higher-butterfat layer skimmed from the top of milk before homogenization

* Half and half (10.5-18% fat) * Light, coffee, or table cream (18-30% fat) * Medium cream (25% fat) * Whipping or light whipping cream (30-36% fat) * Heavy whipping cream (36% or more) * Extra-heavy, double, or manufacturer's cream (38-40% or more)

Source:
http://en.wikipedia.org/wiki/Cream

D.

Deep-fried

Not many cooking rituals are as engrossing to people in most of Europe as deep-frying whole turkeys and all. The food will literally soak up the oil it is cooked in. According to the National Turkey Federation, a 5.9-ounce serving of fried turkey prepared with a dry rub has approximately 383 (19% GDA) calories and 21 grams of fat (30% GDA - 32% RDI). A roast turkey serving has got 362 calories and 16 grams of fat. That's over 30% more fat when deep-fried! This also goes for fish, chicken, steak and whatever more one could imagine throwing in a pot of boiling oil.

Deep-frying is less healthy than baking or grilling, not just because of the oil but the high temperature of the oil will cause it to oxidize (turn rancid) quickly. This is toxic and carcinogenic.

Source:

http://allrecipes.com/Recipe/Deep-Fried-Turkey
http://answers.yahoo.com
http://caloriecount.about.co

Diet-soda

I've had my doubts about diet-soda for a long time. It seems to me that the majority of diet-soda consumers are overweight. I did a little research and found the following:

A study at the University of Texas Health Science Center at San Antonio, reported by Sharon Fowler at the ADA annual meeting, suggests that the consumption of diet soda was correlated with weight gain. Fowler suggested that the undelivered expected calories from diet soda may stimulate the appetite.

"An independent study by researchers with the Framingham Heart Study in Massachusetts has turned up results that indicate that the consumption of diet soda correlates with increased metabolic syndrome. Of the 9,000 males and females studied, findings stated that 48% of the subjects were at higher risk for weight gain and elevated blood sugar. The researchers also acknowledged that diet soda drinkers were less likely to consume healthy foods, and that drinking diet soda flavored with artificial sweeteners more than likely increases cravings for sugar flavored sweets."

Source: wikipedia.org

A Purdue University study released in the journal Behavioral Neuroscience reported that rats on diets containing the artificial sweetener saccharin gained more weight than rats given sugary food, casting doubt on the benefits of low-calorie sweeteners.

Also see Low-sugar and Zero-sugar

Source:
http://abcnews.go.com/GMA/OnCall/story?id=4271246
http://en.wikipedia.org/wiki/Diet_soda

Doggy bags

Another fine example of our cultural differences. Most Europeans would be far too embarrassed to dare to ask to take their leftovers home. "Doggy bags" in the States are so common that some restaurants have custom printed and/or microwavable ones. This correctly implies that restaurant portion sizes are way bigger than a proper meal should be. The meals look like one-size-fits-all meals adapted to the heaviest consumers. It is quite understandable that someone does not want to throw away food he or she has paid for however, smaller size portions wouldn't harm you (or your wallet).

The Wikipedia European sections on "Leftovers" (the few that are there) are generally about making animal food out of it while the US/English section is all about taking leftovers home. That should ring a little bell.

Source:

http://en.wikipedia.org/wiki/Leftovers

Donuts

A policeman's favorite if we should believe the movies. One theory suggests that doughnuts were introduced into North America by Dutch settlers, who were responsible for popularizing other American desserts, including cookies, apple and cream pie.. in the 19th century, doughnuts were sometimes referred to as one kind of olykoek (a Dutch word literally meaning "oil cake/cookie"), a "sweetened cake fried in fat." We call them oliebollen ("oil-balls") and eat them traditionally on New Year. Regional varieties are found throughout the world.

One glazed Dunkin'® donut carries around 180 cal, 8g fat (12% RDI), 1.5g sat. fat (8% RDI), 25g carbs and 6g sugar. Krispy Kreme® adds another 20 cal. Total: 200cal, 12g fat, (18% RDI), 3g sat. fat(15% RDI), 22g carbs and 10g sugar.

One Dutch oliebol has about 140 cal each but we cover them with powdered sugar and eats loads of them! Very unhealthy I might add.

Source:
http://en.wikipedia.org/wiki/Doughnut

Dressing

Let's have a nice light healthy salad one might think. Nothing wrong with that! The dressing is your problem there. A regular serving should be around 2 tbsp (1 oz / 29 g). However, most fast food places will serve you 2 oz packets. A 2 oz packet of ranch dressing contains between 170 and 190 cal, 15 to 20 g of fat (23 to 30% RDI). Caesar dressing adds 20 to 30 cal per packet. Honey-mustard and Thousand Islands go up to 290 cal per 2 oz packet.

Source:
http://caloriecount.about.com
http://nutrition.mcdonalds.com/nutritionexchange/nutritionfacts.pdf

*http://www.bk.com/cms/en/us/cms_out/digital_assets/files/menu_nutrition/Nation
alNutritionals.pdf http://www.whataburger.com/browse_nutritional_info.php*

E.

Eating contests

What should I say? Don't enter them!

See also the Hot Dogs and Steak chapter.

Energy Drinks & Energizers

Energy drinks, shots, bars, chewing gum and what not. Sadly these products have gained enormous popularity over the last 10 years. These products are made to mask fatigue, mask dehydration and use up your natural reserves.

Most energy drinks contain water, sugar, caffeine (often in the form of guarana), taurine or glucuronolactone, vitamin B, minerals, artificial colors and flavors.

One "bullet" can of Red Bull® (250ml or 8.45 fl oz) contains 110 calories, 27 g sugar (30% GDA), 1000 mg taurine, 600 mg glucuronolactone, vitamin B and 80 mg pure caffeine. Monster® energy drink about 100 calories and 27 g of sugar per 8 fl oz. Full Throttle® has 110 calories and 28 g of sugar per 8 fl oz. One 12 fl oz bottle of Gatorade® performance series contains 310 calories and 78 g of carbs (sugars 42 g (42% GDA).

A 2008 position statement issued by the National Federation of State High School Associations made the following recommendations about energy drink consumption, in general, by young athletes:1. Water and appropriate sports drinks should be used for rehydration as outlined in the NFHS Document "Position Statement and Recommendations for Hydration to Minimize the Risk for Dehydration and Heat Illness."2. Energy drinks should not be used for hydration.3. Information about the absence of benefit and the presence of potential risk associated with energy drinks should be widely shared among all individuals who interact with young athletes.4. Energy drinks should not be consumed by athletes who are dehydrated.5. Energy drinks should not be consumed without prior medical approval, by athletes taking over the counter or prescription medications.

In Canada, a can of Red Bull has the following warning on the label: "Caution: Contains caffeine. Not recommended for children, pregnant or breast-feeding women, caffeine sensitive persons or to be mixed with alcohol. Do not consume more than 500ml per day."

Source:

http://caloriecount.about.com

http://en.wikipedia.org/wiki/Red_Bull

http://www.monsterenergy.com

Extra

Extra, extra, eat all about it! The word extra is a statement by itself; unnecessary add-ons! You get it but you don't really need it!

Extra -cheese, -bacon, -mayo, -toppings, -large, anything. Read: Extra -calories, -sugar, -carbs, -salt and -fat!

See also the XL chapter.

F.

Fast food

See Junk Food.

Footlong

Now seriously, a footlong hot dog? A foot long (30 cm -12 inch) sub sandwich? That's like a full dinner meal (and it should be). Here's a couple of examples.

Product	Calories	Fat	Carbs.	Sodium
Dairy Queen® All Beef Foot Long Hot Dog	560	35 g	39 g	1600 mg
RDI	28%	54%	13%	67%
With chilli and cheese	840	54 g	52 g	2050 mg
RDI	42%	69%	17%	85%
Sonics® Extra Long Chilli Cheese Coney	660	39 g	55 g	1860 mg
RDI	33%	60%	18%	78%
Footlong *Subway*® Club	640	10 g	95 g	2320 mg
RDI	32%	15%	32%	97%
Speedway® All American Footlong Sub	821	46.5 g	62 g	3326 mg
RDI	41%	72%	21%	139%

No nutritional info could be found on the Louie's original footlong hot dog.

Also see Sandwiches.

Source:

http://caloriecount.about.com http://www.calorieking.com
http://www.dietfacts.com/html/nutrition-facts
http://www.subway.com/applications/NutritionInfo/nutritionlist.aspx?id=sandwich
http://www.sonicdrivein.com/pdfs/menu/SonicNutritionGuide.pdf

Free Refills

Another thing that hardly anybody believes in my country, free refills! We don't even get free coffee refills in a restaurant! (Yep we are embarrassingly cheap, I guess that's where the idea of "*Going Dutch*" came from) Personally I don't understand why one would pay for a large coke when you can get your small one refilled, free or cheap. I did notice that I had the urge to refill my cup even after I had enough, and found myself drinking more soda than I should or normally would. It's free you know! And I am Dutch.

This is an invitation to consume even more than the incredible sizes served. If you're still thirsty after a 32 fl oz sugared drink, you might want to consider some water.

Fried

See Deep-fried.

Fries

French Fries (poor Belgians, who actually invented fries / frites and are never credited for it) seem to have become one of the Western World's most basic foods. Everybody seems to love them. We, the Dutch, are infamous for "drowning them in mayonnaise" (this is the way they are supposed be consumed according to the Belgians). The quantity has obviously increased during the second half of the 20th Century. Make it - big, extra-large, jumbo, king-size, super-size! Also see the XXL chapter.

In the 1950s, for example, McDonald's original two-ounce serving of fries totaled about 200 calories, but by 2000 the restaurant offered a seven-ounce "super size" sibling that packed 610 calories. It seems that they've gone down to 580 now. Not counting the ketchup or mayo and all the weird high-calorie toppings you have like chili-cheese.

Note: mayonnaise and ketchup are not free in Holland!

The large fries at Burger King® in the US is called king size in the NL.

A little schematic

Burger King© US	Calories	Burger King© NL	Calories
Value Fries	220	Small Fries	203,5
Small	340	Medium	319
Medium	480	Large	390,5
Large	580	King Size	594
McDonalds© US		McDonalds© NL	
Small	230	Small	235
Medium	380	Medium	340
Large	500	Large	470

Makes you wonder why there would be differences at all.

69% of fast-food chains cook their French fries in the unhealthiest oil: corn oil. Corn oil is higher in cholesterol-raising saturated fats than other vegetable oils, a study from the University of Hawaii found. Most restaurants are very hesitant in telling you what they use... McDonalds® lowered their levels of trans fat (oil mix) from 30% to 16% while in Europe 13% to 15% is standard.
Olive oil and Canola oil contain the highest percentage of unsaturated fats and are therefore highly recommended for cooking.
Yes fries are fattening but if cooked properly they're not too bad for a once-a-week treat. A cooking tip: ***French Fries should be fried twice!***

Source:
http://www.bk.com/cms/en/us/cms_out/digital_assets/files/menu_nutrition/NationalNutritionals.pdf
http://www.bloomberg.com/apps/news?pid=20601124&sid=aL3e5kEeyLnI
http://www.burgerking.nl/_content/pdf/bk_nutritions.pdf
http://www.businessweek.com/lifestyle/content/healthday/635088.html
http://www.mcdonaldsmenu.info
http://www.nlm.nih.gov/medlineplus/news/fullstory_94226.html
https://stores.healthmart.com/oakleypharmacy/RelatedItems/6,635088

Fruit Drinks

See Soda-pop / Soft drinks

G.

Giant...

See XXL.

Gravy

What I know as gravy is what Americans call *brown gravy*. It's made from the juices that run naturally from meat while cooking. Red and white gravy are generally unknown outside the US and Canada. Imagine my surprise when I heard someone order biscuits and gravy for the first time!

One Hardee's® biscuit N gravy serving contains over 500 cal. Quite a lot for a side order I thought.

See also the Bicuits and Gravy chapter.

Source:
http://caloriecount.about.com
http://en.wikipedia.org/wiki/Gravy

Grilled

Grilling your food is actually a great low fat cooking choice. The only exception might be grilled cheese sandwiches. Commercial grilled cheese sandwiches run from 280 cal up to 680 cal. A grilled cheese sandwich should be considered a meal, it's not a snack!

Source:
http://caloriecount.about.com

H.

Hamburgers

See Burgers & Beer.

Hot Dogs

Frankfurters, Franks, wieners, wienies, dogs. The perfect Baseball snack I heard! Americans eat a smashing 20 billion (20.000.000.000) hot dogs a year - an average of 70 hot dogs per person! With a peak of 155 million on the 4th of July alone. Estimated by the National Hot Dog & Sausage Council. (Yes, there actually is one!) Nathan's® annual hot dog eating contest 2009 winner ate 68 hot dogs in 10 minutes! With 296.90 calories and 18.21 g of fat per hot dog, that's 8 days worth of calories and over 15 days of fat RDI for a men's 2500 cal diet. (20189.2 calories 1238.28 g - 43.5 oz of fat) Not the smartest of contests to enter I'd say. (That goes for any eating contest for that matter)

The following table shows averages and will differ between restaurants.

Small Hot Dog			Regular Hot Dog		
1.0 oz hot dog bun	2.0 g fat	84 cal	1.5 oz hot dog bun	3.1 g fat	129 cal
Beef frankfurter (5" x 3/4 ", 1.6 oz)	13.3 g fat	149 cal	Beef frankfurter (5" x 7/8 ", 2.0 oz)	16.9 g fat	188 cal
Yellow mustard	0.0 g fat	0 cal	Yellow mustard	0.0 g fat	0 cal
Ketchup (1 tbsp 15g)	0.0 g fat	15 cal	Ketchup (1 tbsp 15g)	0.0 g fat	15 cal
Chili (1/2 cup 31.3 g)	2.4 g fat	40 cal	Chili (1 cup 62.5 g)	4.7 g fat	80 cal
Bacon (strip 8.5 g)	3.0 g fat	40 cal	Bacon (strip 8.5 g)	3.0 g fat	40 cal
Cheese sauce (15g)	1.4 g fat	22 cal	Cheese sauce (28g)	2.8 g fat	43 cal
Cheese (28 g)	9.0 g fat	110 cal	Cheese (28 g)	9.0 g fat	110 cal
Sauerkraut (2.0 oz)	0.0 g fat	13 cal	Sauerkraut (2.0 oz)	0.0 g fat	13 cal
Relish (9 g)	0.0 g fat	10 cal	Relish (9 g)	0.0 g fat	10 cal

The math: A regular chili cheese dog can go up and over 500 calories.

Also see the Footlong chapter.

Source:

http://www.nass.usda.gov
http://hot-dog.org
http://www.nathansfamous.com/FileUpload/File/
09-0217_Nutrition%20Spreadsheet_20080801.pdf
http://caloriecount.about.com
http://www.calorieking.com
http://en.wikipedia.org/wiki/Hot_dog
http://wiki.answers.com

I.

Ice cream

"Everyone likes ice cream no matter who they are" remember the old Sesame Street tune? Thanks Marco Polo for bringing back the 3000 year old recipe. The USA is the world's second leading ice-cream consumer with 5.7 gallons (21.6 liter) per person per year. For comparison: The Dutch and the English consume about 2.1 gallons (8 liter) pp per year.

Scoop sizes are measured in "scoops per quart". A #8 scoop (1/2 cup, 4 oz, 125 ml) will measure 8 scoops per quart; a #10 scoop has 10 scoops per quart. One #8 scoop or 1/2 cup contains about 150 calories, 7.9 g fat and 15.3 g of sugar.

Ice cream may have the following composition: Between 10% and as high as 16% fat in some premium ice creams; 9 to 12% milk solids-not-fat, 12 to 16% sweeteners, 0.2 to 0.5% stabilizers and emulsifiers,â€¨55% to 64% water which comes from the milk or other ingredients.

As mentioned in the documentary film Super Size Me, Ben (Ben & Jerry's) underwent a quintuple bypass in 2001, at the age of 49, to clear blocked arteries, allegedly from ice cream consumption. Burt Baskin (Baskin-Robbins) died of a heart attack at the age of 54. In the documentary Super Size Me, John Robbins attributes his uncle's death and his father's severe diabetes to over consumption of ice cream.

Source:
http://www.wikipedia.com
http://www.dairyinfo.gc.ca
http://www.idfa.org
http://caloriecount.about.com
http://www.calorieking.com

In-betweens

See Snacks Chapter

J.

Jell-O/Jelly

Gelatin: a translucent brittle solid substance, extracted from the collagen inside animal connective tissue. Imagine explaining someone who's never seen Jelly in their life, that this bright and colorful "Never Never Land" - like substance is actually food. I'm sure people would think you're nuts! The radiant colors look so artificial; I'm hesitant to ever try it. The suggested 22 g (0.77 oz) serving size carries 80 cal for the Kraft® gelatin dessert. That's just 1/2 cup friends! If you really feel the urge to eat this, you might want to consider sticking to just that.

Source: http://www.wikipedia.com
http://www.dairyinfo.gc.ca
http://www.idfa.org
http://caloriecount.about.com
http://www.calorieking.com

Jumbo

See XL.

Junk Food

One-third of American diet is junk food and soft drinks. The name itself states exactly what it is: crap food for junkies! Michael Jacobson aptly coins the phrase junk food in 1972 as slang for foods of useless or no nutritional value. Their contents are rich in sodium salts and/or sugar and fats that provide high calories yet useless in value. Easy to prepare and very tasty, sadly enough. People don't want to "waste" time cooking anymore. Question: How can spending time feeding oneself decently (preparing nutritious meals) ever be a waste?

A study by Paul Johnson and Paul Kenny at The Scripps Research Institute suggested that junk food alters brain activity in a manner similar to addictive drugs like cocaine or heroin. Rats addicted to this food would rather starve their selves than eat nutritious food.

Junk Food is a worldwide problem as the bigger franchising companies like McDonalds®, Burger King®, KFC®, Pizza Hut®, Domino's®, Subway® and Starbucks® have expanded their enterprises to almost every country available, and have dominating power over small businesses.

Considering the unavoidable mouth-watering junk food advertising on TV, billboards, magazines, sport events, product placement in movies and TV programs, direction signs and clothing, it's understandable that your mind has gotten used to see this low-grade food it as a "normal" part of your diet. Maybe we should all reconsider that!

Junk Food is the mayor contributor to obesity all over the world!

Here are a couple of frightening facts:

* *At least twenty school districts in the US have their own Subway® franchises; an additional 1,500 districts have Subway contracts; and nine operate Subway sandwich carts.*

* *Taco Bell® sells products in about 4,500 school cafeterias. Pizza Hut®, Domino's Pizza® and McDonald's® are now selling food in US schools. The American School Food Service estimates that about 30 percent of the public high schools in the US offer branded fast food.*

* *Elementary schools in Fort Collins, Colorado now serve food from Pizza Hut, McDonald's and Subway on special lunch days. "We try to be more like the fast food places where these kids are hanging out" a Colorado school administrator told the Denver Post. "We want kids to think school lunch is a cool thing, the cafeteria a cool place, that we're with it."*

* *Pizza Hut, Taco Bell and KFC signed a three-year deal with the National Collegiate Athletic Association. Burger King, Nickelodeon, McDonald's and the Fox Kids Network have formed partnerships that mix advertisements for fast food with children's entertainment. Burger King has sold chicken nuggets shaped like Teletubbies®.*

- Kids who bring their own packed lunch from home are considered "losers".

Source:
http://www.dietpolicy.com/diets-articles/junk-food-facts.htm
http://en.wikipedia.org/wiki/Junk_food
Fast Food Nation: The Dark Side of the All-American Meal - Eric Schlosser
http://www.naturalnews.com/001109.html

K.

King-size

Are you a King? No? Then this is NOT your size!

Also see XL chapter.

KFC

See Fast Food.

Ketchup

It's unbelievable what Americans use ketchup/catsup with; fries, beef, pork, chicken, burgers, hot dogs, beans, sandwiches, soup, eggs, fish, shrimp, salads, potatoes, Mexican food, Spanish food, Italian food (if you want to see a deeply insulted waiter or cook, order ketchup with your spaghetti in Italy), Chinese food. Just about everything you can think of! And it comes free in bulk with all imaginable foods!

Heinz® regards 1 tbsp (17g) to be a serving size, the weird thing is that their new "dip & squeeze" packet design contains 0.95 oz (27 grams). That means you'd have to waste over 33% of the package.

The late former U.S. president Ronald Reagan argued that ketchup is a vegetable because it is red and comes from tomatoes (in attempt to cut balanced lunches funding for school children living in poverty). His wife and First Lady Nancy snapped: "It is not a meat, right? So IT IS a vegetable". This official suggestion was widely ridiculed and the 1981 USDA's proposal was dropped.

Ketchup serving size: 1 Tbsp (17g) Calories: 20, carbs 5g, sugars: 4g (that's one cube per spoon)

Source:

http://www.heinzketchup.com/Products.aspx

http://en.wikipedia.org/wiki/Ketchup
http://www.wikipedia.com

L.

Light

Light... It often means light on one ingredient but not on others. Less fat often means there will be more sugar added and the other way around. Sometimes fat will be replaced by synthetic fat like Olestra which is not absorbed by the body but runs through it and also interferes with the body's absorption of important vitamins, and can cause diarrhea. Light beer can mean lesser calories and just as much alcohol or less alcohol and the same amount of calories.

Also see Low-fat and Nonfat.

Source:
http://www.fitsugar.com
http://www.wikipedia.com

Low-fat

Low-fat does NOT mean low-calories! Many low-fat foods have loads of sugar as substitute and to give them some taste. Low-fat means there should be no more than 3g of fat per serving.

A major misconception in the US seems to be that all fats are bad for you, or that you don't need them in your diet. You do! Fat is necessary for the absorption of fat-soluble vitamins A, D, E and K, for proper neurological function, healthy skin and hair, protecting vital organs, to help keep us warm and for pleasure (endorphins). Diets too low in fat (less than 20 - 25%) may trigger cravings. Fat is not the biggest cause of obesity, carbohydrates are (sugars).

See also Nonfat and Sugar.

Source:
http://www.eatingdisordersonline.com/nutritional/fats.php

http://lowfatcooking.about.com/od/lowfatbasics/tp/fatfallacies.htm
http://wiki.answers.com/Q/What_is_the_difference_between_regular_and_low_fat_fo
ods
http://www.wikipedia.com

Low-sugar

Low-sugar does NOT per definition mean low-calories either! Low on sugar often means high on fat. Read the Nutrition Facts on your products!

See also Sugar and Zero-sugar.

M.

Macaroni & Cheese / Meatballs & Spaghetti

Macaroni & Cheese is NOT a dish, nor should it be! I've read a website mentioning the history of cooking mac & cheese, talking about the recipe being cooked this way for over 500 years. NO! Macaroni & Cheese is not an Italian dish, neither is Meatballs & Spaghetti. Yes you get cheese on top of the pasta-sauce on your macaroni, but not just cheese. Just look at a bowl of it, it looks gross, be real! I've shown pictures of mac "n cheese to people here in The Netherlands, and no-one can believe that you guys really eat this. Kraft® mac and cheese dinners(?!) were introduced to the US in 1937 and now everybody actually believes this is a real Italian meal. It's a snack, guys! Check the Food Pyramid, what are we missing here? Vegies, meat-beans-nuts, fruits? Vitamins?

1 serving of Kraft® Macaroni & Cheese Dinner is based on 1 cup, NOT a bowl! Remember that next time you grab the box. There's 240 cal, 8g fat, 4g sat. fat, 34g carbs, 10g sugar in that cup.

I've seen Americans go into Italian restaurants in Italy, and making fools of themselves by getting annoyed because Meatballs & Spaghetti or Macaroni & Cheese are not on the menu. (Not even mentioning the ketchup you want along with everything to ruin all flavors, which is an insult to any Chef I must add). In fact I've been in Italian Delis in the States without even a single authentic Italian meal on the menu.

Source:
http://healthylivingtools.kraftfoods.com
http://www.macaronicheeserecipes.com/Macaroni-and-Cheese-History.htm
http://en.wikipedia.org/wiki/Macaroni_and_cheese

Mayonnaise

I know the Dutch are famous for "drowning our fries in Mayonnaise" (John Travolta in Pulp Fiction) but Americans sure know their way around it too. 48 and 64 oz jars? That's begging for over-usage. The Dutch don't even have these (and that's saying something) nor would anyone here buy them I'm sure, fast food restaurants excluded. I've hardly ever seen any sandwich that wasn't heavily spread with mayo, (We use a thin layer of butter)

Ever noticed that low-fat mayo has 2 or 3 times more sugar than regular mayo?

McDonald's

See Junk Food.

Milkshakes

I remember the first large milkshake I ever had at some fast food restaurant well. Large it was, 44 oz (1.3 ltr) a third of a gallon (r u 4 real?). Being Dutch (and human), I couldn't finish half the thing but I felt uneasy throwing it away. A large McDonald's shake in the Netherlands is 16.9 oz (0.5 ltr) that should be plenty for anyone. And if you're still thirsty, you might wanna try some water!

In the 40's and 50's, milkshakes were served in 12 1/2-ounce tall, "y"-shaped glasses, a very reasonable size for a delicious but extremely high-calorie treat! Nowadays we can't seem to get enough of it.

Here we go:

Product	Serving Size	Calories	Carbs.	Sugar(*)	Fat	Protein
Burger King® Chocolate Milk Shake	32oz (0.95 ltr)	990	178 g	171 g	31 g	17 g
RDI		49.5%	59%	190%	48%	34%
Jack In The Box® Chocolate Shake with Whipped Topping	24 oz (0.71 ltr)	1150	146 g	128 g	55 g	19 g
RDI		57.5%	49%	142%	84%	47%
McDonalds® Chocolate Triple Thick® Shake	32 oz (0.95 ltr)	1160	203 g	168 g	27 g	27 g
RDI		58%	68%	187%	42%	47%
Whataburger® large shake	44 oz (1.3 ltr)	1380	242 g	222 g	36 g	31 g
RDI		69%	81%	247%	55%	62%
And if that isn't crazy enough for you, here's the current record holder:						
White Castle® Chocolate Shake Louisville region	44 oz (1.3 ltr)	1680	277 g	211 g	48 g	35 g
RDI		84%	92%	234%	74%	70%
* Percentage in GDA since there is no RDI for sugar						

That's just way too much for one drink people, these sizes should be outlawed for health's sake. Even a kid's shake covers 89% of your daily sugar intake. Wake up folks! No one person needs that. This is far beyond ridiculous!

It needs to be said, some fast-food restaurants keep reasonable large sizes nowadays: Denny's® 16oz, Sonics® 20oz.

Source:
http://www.bk.com/cms/en/us/cms_out/digital_assets/files/pages/NationalNutritio nals.pdf http://www.dennys.com/LiveImages/enProductImage_790.pdf
http://en.wikipedia.org/wiki/Milkshake
http://www.jackinthebox.com/pdf/NutritionalGuide_2010.pdf
http://nutrition.mcdonalds.com/nutritionexchange/nutritionfacts.pdf
http://www.sonicdrivein.com/pdfs/menu/SonicNutritionGuide.pdf
http://www.whataburger.com/browse_nutritional_info.php
http://www.whitecastle.com/system/blocks/data/6/original/20091208_wc_nutrition .pdf

N.

Nachos

Tortilla chips or nachos are made from corn tortillas (corn, vegetable oil, salt and water) cut into wedges and fried. I was amazed to find that 1 serving size of 11 nacho chips could contain 140 cal. Dip "m in salsa (4 cal per tbsp), sour cream (26 cal per tbsp) guacamole (36 cal per tbsp). On a platter with meat, beans, chili and cheese, micro waved and topped with jalapeños, olives and what not. An appetizer? Sounds like a full meal.

Product	Serving Size	Calories	Fat	Carbs.	Sodium
Doritos® Nacho Cheese	11 nachos 1oz/28.3g	140	8 g	17 g	180 mg
RDI		7%	12%	6%	8%
Taco Bell® Nachos	3.4oz/98g	320	31 g	32 g	530 mg
RDI		16%	31%	11%	22%
Nachos with Cheese	6-8 nachos 4oz/113g	346	19 g	37 g	816 mg
RDI		17%	29%	12%	34%
Taco John's® Chicken Super Nachos	12.3oz/350g	780	45 g	62 g	2250 mg
RDI		39%	69%	21%	94%

See also Potato Chips.

Source:

http://caloriecount.about.com
http://en.wikipedia.org/wiki/Nachos
http://en.wikipedia.org/wiki/Tortilla_chips

Nonfat

Nonfat does not per definition mean NO FAT nor NO CALORIES! Yes, I know it should! But corporate business has created all sorts of legal tricks to mislead you, all for the economy and greedy stockholders" wallets (and if you are one, shame on you!). Of course you can label candy, loaded with sugar and carbs, "Fat-Free" but why would you, if not to mislead? A dollar is more important than honesty and people's health it seems... No(n) Fat or fat free means less than 0.5 grams of fat per serving.

Here's a list of some Nonfat products, note the high sugar percentages:

Nonfat products	Size	Calories	Fat	Carbs.	Sugar (*)
Milk	1 cup (245g)	86	0.4 g	12.3 g	12.3 g
RDI			4.3%	0.6%	4.1%	13.6%
Frozen Yoghurt (TCBY®)	1/2 cup (98g)	110	0.0 g	23.0 g	20.0 g
RDI			5.5%	0%	7.7%	22%
Mayonnaise (Ruby's Diner®)	1 1/2 tbsp (22g)	17	1.0 g	3.0 g	2.0 g
RDI			0.9%	1.5%	1%	2.2%
Ice Cream (Edy's®)	1/4 cup (61g)	90	0.0 g	20.0 g	4.0 g
RDI			4.5%	0%	6.7%	4.4%
French Vanilla Creamer (H.E.B.®)	1 tbsp (15g)	35	2.0 g	6.0 g	5.0 g
RDI			1.8%	3%	2%	5.6%
* Percentage in GDA since there is no RDI for sugar					

See also Low-Fat.

Source:
http://en.wikipedia.org/wiki/
http://caloriecount.about.com
http://www.livestrong.com/thedailyplate/

O.

Obesity

Globally there are more than 300 million obese adults; over 72 million of them are Americans!

Obesity is a condition where you body-mass-index (BMI) is greater than 30 kg/m2 according to the W.H.O. You are overweight when your BMI is between 25 and 30 kg/m2. (mass(LB) x 4.88 / height(FT)2) National Center for Health Statistics shows the number of obese Americans now outweighing the number of overweight Americans, 33.8% to 32.7% (while 40 million Americans will need food handouts/help this year). That means that only one in three Americans could be considered healthy.

Obesity is the #2 cause of preventable death in the United States. The list of chronic physical and mental illnesses associated with obesity is endless, here's a handful: heart failure, COPD, cellulites, diabetes, erectile dysfunction, high blood pressure, infertility, migraines, sleep apnea.

It also needs to be pointed out that overweight or obese parents, often unintentionally, tend to overfeed their children (and pets). I hereby vote for mandatory food and health education in all schools, and to ban all junk food restaurants from serving food at schools.

Note: During my research, I couldn't help but notice the striking parallel between the increasing number of obese people and the decreasing number of smokers in the USA. I certainly do not want to promote smoking but the data is remarkable. Adult smokers percentage went down from 42% in 1965 to 21% in 2004, adult obesity went up from 14% to 34% in the same period. I would like to see some research on the correlation.

Source:
http://www.getamericafit.org/statistics-obesity-in-america.html
http://www.cdc.gov/nchs/data/databriefs/db01.pdf

http://www.cdc.gov/obesity/data/trends.html
http://en.wikipedia.org/wiki/Obesity
http://en.wikipedia.org/wiki/Obesity_associated_morbidity
http://www.newsbatch.com/tob-smokprev1.html
http://www.reuters.com/article/idUSTRE50863H20090109

http://www.who.int/dietphysicalactivity/publications/facts/obesity/en/

Over-consumption

Whether it is salt, sugar, carbs or fat, over-consumption leads to obesity. Overdoing anything is never very healthy! We've been led to believe that the oversized portions served in restaurants nowadays are "normal sizes". Billboards, TV, Newspaper advertisements are so cleverly constructed, they can be irresistibly mouthwatering just to look at. Cheap too! So what's keeping you?

40 to 50% of all edible foods in the US are wasted! (According to a study by the University of Arizona.) Whole batches of perfectly drinkable soft drinks are destroyed for having a crooked or misprinted label, restaurants throw away what they don't use, we don't finish our immense plates and let products expire, supermarkets are forced to throw away any fruit or veggie with a little blemish on them (try growing your own apples without a spot here and there). We all became too spoiled, having the choice to pick them out ourselves, not thinking about the cost of the ones that have to be discarded, subsequently raising the prices. Imagine, you could literally feed Ethiopia, South Africa and Somalia with this "waste".

Human demand on the Earth's ecosystems is measured in Ecological Footprint. In 2006 humanity's total ecological footprint was estimated at 1.4 planet Earths, meaning we used 1.4 more that the earth could renew. You can (should) calculate your own personal footprint on one of these websites (beware, this can be shocking!):

- http://footprint.wwf.org.uk

- http://www.myfootprint.org

- http://www.footprintnetwork.org
- http://www.carbonfootprint.com

Source:
http://www.ers.usda.gov/publications/foodreview/jan1997/jan97a.pdf
http://en.wikipedia.org/wiki/Ecological_footprint
http://uanews.org/node/10448

Overeating

Ye olde Christmas holidays feeling after overindulging in a feast. "More for Less!" It needs to be said that going out for dinner is a lot cheaper in the USA than it is here in The Netherlands, and I mean a lot cheaper! And again, as the portions are so incredibly huge, it's very tempting to eat "till you're stuffed (and kid yourself into thinking that the meal size was proportional). When you overeat, you cause your stomach to expand and force it to be able to accept more food next time.

Compulsive overeaters, food addicts, spend excessive amounts of time and thought devoted to food, and secretly plan or fantasize about eating alone. This is treatable with counseling and therapy.

Also see the All You Can Eat... and (Footlong) Hot Dogs chapters.

Source:
http://en.wikipedia.org/wiki/Overeating
http://en.wikipedia.org/wiki/Compulsive_overeating

Oversized

See XXL.

P.

Pancakes

The first time I saw the stacks of pancakes covered with syrup was in a cartoon. I thought it was a joke but I later found, to my surprise, that you guys really do eat whole stacks of flapjacks. To us "Old World folks", it looks like you misinterpreted the idea of stacking pancakes. We stack"m in the middle of the dining table so the whole family can take one thin pancake, eat it and then take another. With the exception of Australia and the US, I have found no other countries where people eat whole stacks per person!

Product	Calories	Fat	Carbs.	Sodium
One average pancake	110	3g (5%)	11g (6%)	470mg (19%)
One serving of syrup - 1/4 cup (60g)	210	0g	52g (17%)	120mg (5%)
One serving of butter - 1 tbsp (14g)	100	11g (17%)	0g	95mg (4%)

Percentages R.D.I. according to the F.D.A.

Some companies still don't publish nutritional data. Personally I think that publishing nutritional data should be the law!

Here are a couple of breakfast menus (oversized diner meals) you should consider skipping:

Product	Serving Size	Calories	Fat	Carbs.	Sodium
Denny's®					
2 Breakfast Pancakes	6oz, 170g	340	4 g	68 g	1180 mg
RDI		17%	6%	23%	49%
3 side Pancakes buttermilk	9oz, 255g	510	6 g	102 g	1770 mg
RDI		26%	9%	34%	74%
Fruit-Filled Pancakes Blueberry *	18oz, 510g	921	55 g	74 g	2430 mg
RDI		46%	85%	25%	101%
* *contains 530mg chol (177%)*					
IHOP®					
Double Blueberry Pancakes	4 pancakes	800	17 g	115 g	700 mg
RDI		40%	26%	38%	29%
Kids Funny Face Pancake	2 pancakes	1456	69 g	77 g	556 mg
RDI		73%	06%	26%	23%
Shoney's®					
Pancake Platter	Half Stack	932	14 g	187 g	2592 mg
RDI		47%	21%	62%	108%
Pancake platter	Deluxe	1609	32 g	299 g	4988 mg
RDI		80%	50%	100%	208%

Source:
http://www.dennys.com/LiveImages/enProductImage_790.pdf
http://en.wikipedia.org/wiki/Pancake
http://www.livestrong.com
http://www.slimkicker.com

Pie

There are many kinds but the most famous pie must be Dutch apple pie. I guess it makes us Dutchmen "guilty" for bringing it to the US. Granny's recipe, great with whipped cream! Here's a list with nutrition for apple pie from some well known fast food restaurants:

Product	Serving Size	Calories	Carbs.	Sugar(*)	Fat	Sat. Fat
Subway® Apple Pie	1 pie (71 g)	245	37 g	25 g	10 g	2 g
RDI		12%	12%	28%	15%	10%
McDonalds® Baked Hot Apple Pie	1 pie (77 g)	250	32 g	13 g	13 g	7 g
RDI		13%	11%	14%	20%	35%
Burger King® Dutch Apple Pie	1 pie (107 g)	320	46 g	23 g	14 g	6 g
RDI		16%	15%	25%	22%	30%
Shoney's® Apple Nutrasweet Pie	1 serving	454	64 g	32 g	18 g	4 g
RDI		23%	21%	35%	28%	20%
Denny's® Apple Pie	1 serving	470	64 g	36 g	24 g	6 g
RDI		24%	21%	40%	37%	30%
Percentage in GDA since there is no RDI for sugar						

Source:
http://caloriecount.about.com

Pizza

By far the most considered food when one doesn't feel like cooking! Approximately 3 billion pizzas per year are sold in the USA. Front door delivery for the lazy folks so you won't have to burn a single calorie to get one. Wikipedia states that: "Pizza is an oven-baked, flat, disc-shaped bread typically topped with a tomato sauce, cheese (usually mozzarella) and various toppings depending on the culture... the US has developed regional forms of pizza, some bearing only a casual resemblance to the Italian original."

Calories, calories calories!!! It's just incredible how the US food industry managed to turn this into one of the most fattening foods on the planet. The bigger, the better. Loads of salt. Cheese everywhere, even in the crust! Toppings like pineapple that would make any Italian roll their eyes. And cheap (in every definition of the word)!

Product	Serving Size	Calories	Fat	Carbs.	Sodium
Domino's®					
Classic Pepperoni 14" Pizza	1 slice (1/8)	324	13 g	39 g	608 mg
RDI	(120 g)	16%	19%	13%	25%
Papa John's®					
Pepperoni 14" Pizza	1 slice (1/8)	330	14 g	37 g	870 mg
RDI	(130 g)	17%	22%	12%	36%
Pizza Hut®					
Large Pan Pepperoni 14" pizza	1 slice (1/8)	380	19 g	36 g	840 mg
RDI	(128 g)	19%	29%	12%	35%
Large Pan Meatlovers® 14" pizza	1 slice (1/8)	480	28 g	37 g	1180 mg
RDI	(160 g)	24%	45%	12%	49%

Everybody enjoys a pizza every once in a while, but keep the portions in mind; a whole pizza can easily hold 100% carbs, over 2 times your fat RDI and more than 3 times your daily salt.

You should try to make your own pizza, it's very easy and a lot of fun to do and healthier too. I bet you'll wonder what you've been paying for all this time.

Source:

http://en.wikipedia.org/wiki/Pizza
http://www.divinecaroline.com/79975/49492-portion-size-vs-now

http://www.dominos.com/home/menu/nutrition.jsp
http://www.my-personaltrainer.it/nutrizione/calorie-pizza.html
http://www.papajohns.com/menu/nutritional_info.shtm

http://www.pizzahut.com/nutrition.aspx

http://www.pizzaware.com/facts.htm
http://www.nutritiondata.com

Potato-Chips

I deliberately left out potatoes as a fattener because they are not by themselves! (I heard Oprah warn about their calories). It's how you prepare/eat them. Boiled potatoes contain about 110 cal per 150g/5.3oz, (that's less than white rice and noodles, i.e. 190 and 200 per 150g) mashed potatoes 125 cal and French fries about 320 cal per 150g. That's nothing compared to potato chips!

Potato chips; US serving size: 1oz/28g, that's 12 chips! Europe: 0.88oz/25g, 11 chips. 12 chips per serving size, I honestly never thought it was that little.

Product	Serving Size	Calories	Fat	Carbs.	Sodium
Lays® Classic	1oz/12 chips	150	10 g	15g	180mg
RDI			7%	15%	5%	8%
Pringles® Original	1oz/14 chips	160	11g	14g	170mg
RDI			8%	17%	5%	7%

Americans eat over $6 billion worth of potato-chips a year.

Source:

http://caloriecount.about.com

http://www.lifeintheusa.com/food/snackfoods.htm
http://www.livestrong.com

Q.

Quarter Pounder

See Burgers & Beer

Quesadillas

It never ceases to amaze me how a small sandwich-like thing can pack so many calories. Two tortillas with melted cheese in between, sure doesn't sound like a fat-bomb, yet it can be.

Product	Serving Size	Calories	Fat	Carbs.	Sodium
Taco Bell®					
Cheese quesadilla	142 g	470	26 g	40 g	1120mg
RDI		24%	40%	13%	47%
Chicken quesadilla	184 g	520	28 g	41 g	1440mg
RDI		26%	43%	14%	60%
Taco Bueno®					
Cheese quesadilla	185 g	709	42 g	48 g	1261 mg
RDI		35%	65%	16%	53%
Chicken quesadilla:	225g	761	44 g	50g	1658mg
RDI		38%	68%	17%	69%
Taco Del Mar®					
Cheese quesadilla:	282g	710	54 g	63 g	990 mg
RDI		35%	43%	21%	41%
Beef quesadilla:	353g	800	37 g	66 g	1540 mg
RDI		40%	57%	22%	64%
California Tortilla®					
Cheese quesadilla:	182g	594	32 g	48 g	863 mg
RDI		30%	49%	16%	36%
Chicken quesadilla:	273g	723	35 g	49 g	1407 mg
RDI		36%	53%	16%	59%
Chicken quesadilla Lite:	273g	615	21 g	48 g	1191 mg
RDI		31%	32%	16%	50%
Applebee's®					
"Low Fat" chicken quesadilla:	1 serving	742	14 g	89 g	?mg
RDI		37%	22%	30%	?%

Source:
http://www.applebees.com/downloads/Applebees_Nutritional_Info.pdf
http://caloriecount.about.com/
http://www.livestrong.com/

http://nutrition.californiatortilla.com/recipe_categories.php

http://www.tacobell.com/nutrition/information
http://www.tacobueno.com/nutrition/
http://www.tacodelmar.com/food/nutrition.html

R.

Ribs

Why would any food producer create unhealthy products with portions that exceed your Recommended Daily Values? Why do we allow them to do it? Any restaurant serving size of ribs seems to be guilty of this. Check out these calories, fat and salt contents and ask yourself: "Do I really need this?"

Product	Calories	Fat	Carbohydrates	Sodium
Applebees®				
Double-Glazed Baby Back Ribs	1240 - 1460	73 - 75 g	87 - 129 g	2530 - 3650 mg
RDI	62 - 73%	**112 - 115**%	29 - 43%	**101 - 152**%
Riblets Platter	1570 - 1700	87 - 88 g	100 - 130 g	4010 - 5650 mg
RDI	79 - 85%	**134 - 135**%	33 - 43%	**167 - 235**%
Chilis®				
Original Ribs - Full Rack	1110	81 g	33 g	4100 mg
RDI	62 - 73%	**125**%	11%	**171**%
Outback Steakhouse®				
Baby Back Ribs - Full Rack	1582	113.8 g	23.4 g	2631 mg
RDI	79%	**175**%	8%	**109**%

The "world famous" Waldo's® does not publish nutritional information.

Source:
http://www.applebees.com/downloads/Applebees_Nutritional_Info.pdf
http://caloriecount.about.com/
http://www.chilisnutrition.com/
http://www.livestrong.com/
http://www.outback.com/menu/nutritionselection.aspx

S.

Sugar

Rebelling against alphabetic order I need to start this chapter with the unavoidable, unequalled, unregulated and by far the most addictive drug mankind has ever known: sugar! Over 75% of the world is a sugar junkie!

THERE's SUGAR IN ALMOST EVERYTHING!!

Sugar: an informal term for a class of edible crystalline carbohydrates, mainly sucrose (table sugar), lactose (sugar in milk), and fructose (fruit sugar) characterized by a sweet flavor. (*)

Your parents have unknowingly started your addiction to it with the first Baby Formula you ever had. And since we eat and drink sugary foods almost constantly, we keep on feeding our addiction. The average American consumes around 160 pounds of sugar each year, that's about an average American woman's full weight in sugar. Milk, tomato sauce, salad dressing, soup, crackers, even a can of peas (actually all canned vegetables) has sugar added because the "taste-tests" showed people found them nicer with sugar than plain. Peas with added sugar, I ask you!? Lipton® goes as far as to put additional sugar in their teabags as "flavoring" without listing it as ingredient.

When sugar enters the bloodstream, blood sugar levels rise, causing the pancreas to release insulin. Insulin converts sugar into energy and fat, giving you a "high". When the glucose is gone from your blood, you "crash". This can cause addiction-like behavior.

Sugar releases the same craving-triggering opioids in the brain as heroin and morphine do.

Tooth decay, obesity, diabetes, depressed immune system, hyperactivity, high blood pressure, epileptic seizures, depression, migraine, heart disease, various cancers, multiple sclerosis and many more medical conditions could be related to sugar intake.

The Domino Sugar Company has established the following volume to weight conversions:

Brown sugar 1 cup = 48 teaspoons ~ 195 g = 6.88 oz = 194.66 g carbs
Granular sugar 1 cup = 48 teaspoons ~ 200 g = 7.06 oz = 199.6 g carbs
Powdered sugar 1 cup = 48 teaspoons ~ 120 g = 4.23 oz = 119.6 g carbs

Added Sugar

Added sugar contributes nothing but calories and is therefore known as "dead food". Natural whole foods are a contributor of nutrients, while dead foods are users of nutrients. There is added sugar in anything from candy, cake, cookies, ice-cream, soft drinks and fruit juice to bread, canned vegetables, deli meat, ketchup, soup and many more foods.

Hidden Sugar

We call sugar "hidden sugar" when the ingredients on the label do not use the word sugar and try to mislead you into thinking the product is healthier than is actually is. (Yes, there should be a law against this!) Food companies will do everything to confuse you regarding added/hidden sugars. They often don't want you to realize how much sugar is used in their products and will try to hide the truth from you by using different names on the labels. Sugar is a very cheap filler and preservative ingredient and makes your brain think the product tastes nice. Lipton® for instance goes as far as calling it aroma so the don't have to refer to sugar at all.

Names for added/hidden sugars on food labels:

* Agave nectar (Often with HFCS)

* Agave syrup (Often with HFCS

* All natural evaporated cane juice

* Amasake

* Amber liquid sugar

* Anhydrous dextrose

* Apple butter (Usually with HFCS)

* Apple fructose

* Apple sugar

* Apple syrup

* Arenga sugar

* Azucar morena

* Bakers special sugar

* Barbados Sugar

* Barley malt

* Barley malt syrup

* Bar sugar

* Berry Sugar

* Beet molasses

* Beet sugar

* Beet sugar molasses

* Beet syrup

* Birch syrup

* Blackstrap molasses

* Blonde coconut sugar

* Brown rice syrup

* Brown sugar

* Buttered syrup

* Candy floss

* Candy syrup

* Candi syrup

* Cane crystals

* Cane juice

* Cane juice crystals

* Cane juice powder

* Cane sugar

* Caramel

* Carob syrup

* Caster sugar

* Castorsugar

* Cellobiose

* Chicory (HFCS)

* Coarse sugar

* Coconut nectar

* Coconut palm sugar

* Coconut sap sugar

* Coconut sugar

* Coconut syrup

* Coco sugar

* Coco sap sugar

* Concentrate juice (Often with HFCS)

* Concord grape juice concentrate (Often with HFCS)

* Confectioner's sugar

* Corn sugar (HFCS)

* Corn syrup (may contain some HFCS)

* Corn syrup powder (may contain some HFCS)

* Corn syrup solids (may contain some HFCS)

* Corn sweetener (HFCS)

* Cornsweet ® (really HFCS 90)

* Creamed honey (Often with HFCS)

* Crystal dextrose

* Crystalline fructose

* Crystallized organic cane juice

* Crystal sugar

* D-arabino-hexulose

* Dark brown sugar

* Dark molasses

* Date sap

* Date sugar

* Decorating sugar

* Dehydrated sugar cane juice

* Demerara sugar

* Demerara light sugar

* Dextrin

* Dextran

* Dextrose

* D-fructose

* D-fructofuranose

* D-glucose

* Diastatic malt

* Diatase

* Disaccharide

* Dixie crystals

* D-mannose

* Dried corn syrup

* Dried evaporated organic cane juice

* D-xylose

* ECJ

* Evaporated organic cane juice

* Evaporated corn sweetener (HFCS)

* Ethyl maltol

* First molasses

* Florida Crystals

* Free Flowing

* Free flowing brown sugar

* Fructamyl

* Fructosan (may contain HFCS)

* Fructose (HFCS)

* Fructose crystals (HFCS)

* Fructose sweetener (HFCS)

* Fruit fructose (HFCS)

* Fruit juice (Often with HFCS)

* Fruit juice concentrate (Often with HFCS)

* Fruit sugar (Often with HFCS)

* Fruit syrup (Often with HFCS)

* Galactose

* Glucodry

* Glucomalt

* Glucoplus

* Glucose

* Glucose-fructose syrup (HFCS)

* Glucose solids

* Glucose syrup

* Glucosweet

* Gluctose fructose (HFCS)

* Golden molasses

* Golden sugar

* Golden syrup (GMO beet)

* Gomme syrup

* Granulated coconut nectar

* Granulated coconut sugar

* Granulated fructose

* Granulated sugar

* Granulated sugar cane juice

* Granulized cane sugar

* Grape sugar

* Grape juice concentrate (Often with HFCS)

* Gur

* HFCS

* HFCS 42

* HFCS 55

* HFCS 90

* High dextrose glucose syrup

* High-fructose corn syrup

* High fructose maize syrup (HFCS)

* High maltose corn syrup (Often with HFCS)

* Hydrogenated starch

* Hydrogenated starch hydrolysate

* Hydrolyzed corn starch (Often with HFCS)

* Honey

* Honey comb

* Honey powder

* HSH

* Icing sugar

* Inulin (HFCS)

* Invert sugar

* Inverted sugar

* Inverted sugar syrup

* Invert syrup

* Icing sugar

* Isoglucose (HFCS)

* Isomalt

* Isomaltotriose

* Isosweet

* Jaggery

* Jaggery powder

* Lactitol

* Lactose

* Levulose

* Lesys

* Light brown sugar

* Light molasses

* Liquid dextrose

* Liquid fructose (Often with HFCS)

* Liquid fructose syrup (Often with HFCS)

* Liquid honey (Often with HFCS)

* Liquid maltodextrin

* Liquid sucrose

* Liquid sugar

* Maize sugar

* Maize syrup (HFCS)

* Maldex

* Maldexel

* Malt

* Malted barley syrup HFCS)

* Malted corn syrup (HFCS)

* Malted corn and barley syrup (HFCS

* Malted barley

* Maltitol

* Maltitol syrup

* Malitsorb

* Maltisweet

* Maltodextrin

* Maltose

* Maltotriitol

* Maltotriose

* Maltotriulose

* Malt syrup

* Mannitol

* Maple Sugar

* Maple syrup (Sometimes with HFCS)

* Meritose

* Meritab 700

* Milk sugar

* Misri

* Mizuame

* Molasses

* Molasses sugar

* Monosaccharide

* Morena

* Muscovado sugar

* Mycose

* Mylose

* Nigerotriose

* Nipa sap

* Nipa syrup

* Oligosaccharide

* Organic agave syrup

* Organic brown rice syrup

* Organic cane juice crystals

* Organic coconut nectar

* Organic coconut sugar

* Organic coconut palm sugar

* Organic granulated coconut sugar

* Organic maple syrup

* Organic palm sugar

* Organic rice syrup

* Organic sucanat

* Organic sugar

* Organic raw sugar

* Orgeat syrup

* Palm sap

* Palm sugar

* Palm syrup

* Panela

* Pancake syrup (Often with HFCS)

* Panocha

* Pearl sugar

* Piloncillo

* Potato maltodextrine

* Potato syrup

* Powdered sugar

* Promitor

* Pure fructose crystals (HFCS)

* Pure cane syrup

* Pure sugar spun

* Raisin syrup

* Rapadura

* Raw agave syrup

* Raw sugar

* Raffinose

* Refiner's syrup (Often with HFCS)

* Rice bran syrup

* Rice malt

* Rice maltodextrine

* Rice malt syrup

* Rice syrup

* Rice syrup solids

* Raw honey

* Rock sugar

* Saccharose

* Sanding sugar

* Second molasses

* Shakar

* Simple syrup (Often with HFCS)

* Sirodex

* Soluble corn fiber

* Sorbitol

* Sorbitol syrup

* Sorghum

* Sorghum molasses

* Sorghum syrup

* Sucanat

* Sucre de canne naturel

* Sucrose

* Sucrosweet

* Sugar

* Sugar beet syrup

* Sugar beet crystals

* Sugar beet molasses

* Sugar cane juice

* Sugar cane natural

* Sugar glass

* Sugar hat

* Sugar pine

* Sulfured molasses

* Sweetened condensed milk (Often with HFCS)

* Sweet sorghum syrup

* Syrup Syrup

* Table sugar

* Taffy

* Tagatose

* Tapioca syrup

* Toddy

* Treacle

* Trehalose

* Tremalose

* Trimoline

* Triose

* Trisaccharides

* Turbinado sugar

* Unrefined sugar

* Unsulphured molasses

* Wheat syrup

* White crystal sugar

* White grape juice concentrate (Often with HFCS)

* White refined sugar

* White sugar

* Wood sugar

* Xylose

* Yacon syrup

* Yellow sugar

High Fructose Corn Syrup - H.F.C.S.

See Syrup

No Sugar added

I understand how this can be very misleading. You would think you're getting something healthy and natural right? Wrong! No sugar added just means no additional sugar from anything but the product. You can put as much apple-sugar in apple-juice as you want and still officially sell it as 100% juice, no sugar added!

Also see Syrup.

Source:
* Definition by Wikipedia
http://www.bupa.co.uk/health_information/html/health_news/190703addic.html
http://www.cbsnews.com/stories/2004/03/19/earlyshow/saturday/main607396.sht ml

http://en.wikipedia.org/wiki/Sugar

http://en.wikipedia.org/wiki/Sugar_addiction
http://ezinearticles.com/?Sugar---What-Happens-When-You-Eat-It?&id=4144360
https://www.facebook.com/notes/single-mans-kitchen/all-the-249-names-of-sugar-so-far-project/10150839799498198
http://health.usnews.com/health-news/diet-fitness/articles/2009/08/24/foods-surprisingly-high-in-added-sugar.html
http://www.hookedonjuice.com/
http://www.mypyramid.gov/pyramid/discretionary_calories_sugars.htmlhttp://natural healthperspective.com/food/sugar.html
http://rheumatic.org/sugar.htm
http://uk.askmen.com/sports/foodcourt_150/153_eating_well.html
http://www.usda.gov/factbook/chapter2.pdf

Salt

The average American consumes twice the Recommended Daily Intake of salt, 50% more than in the 1980's. The United States Department of Health and Human Service and the American Heart Association recommend salt consumption of 2,400mg, about one teaspoon, a day.

Salt is not the same as sodium. Table salt is made up of 40% sodium and 60% chloride. We need salt to maintain all body fluids at an optimum level. Consuming too much salt can cause fluids to be retained in the body tissues, causing heart disorders and high blood pressure.

Obesity, stroke, cardiovascular disease, high blood pressure, kidney disease, cardiac enlargement, edema (oedema), duodenal and gastric ulcers, heartburn, osteoporosis, premenstrual syndrome and stomach cancer are medical conditions related to excess salt intake. The intake of large amounts of salt (1g per kg bodyweight) in a short time can result in death.

High salt foods are: bread, canned vegetables, cereals, cheese, fast food (burger, fries, pancakes, pizza), processed meat (sausages, bacon, ham, luncheon meat), (pasta) sauces, snacks (potato chips, pretzels), soups.

Excess salt intake also leads to an urge to consume more sugary soft drinks.

If you want to lose weight, eat less salt!

Source:
http://www.dummies.com/how-to/content/lowering-your-salt-intake.html
http://en.wikipedia.org/wiki/Salt
http://www.eurekalert.org/pub_releases/2006-11/uoh-sii110106.php#
http://www.fatfreekitchen.com/nutrition/high-sodium.html
http://www.hs.fi/english/article/Finnish+study+links+heavy+salt+intake+with+ob
esity/1135222731879 http://msds.chem.ox.ac.uk/SO/sodium_chloride.html
http://news.softpedia.com/news/Salt-Consumption-Connected-to-Obesity-Risk-
40099.shtml http://www.ncbi.nlm.nih.gov/pubmed/12113591
http://www.safeslimming.co.uk/SaltAndSodium.html
http://www.wndu.com/mmm/headlines/16362456.html

Sandwiches

Every time I make myself a sandwich in the US, someone will tell me not to be shy with the deli-meat. One or maybe two slices of luncheon meat per sandwich is enough for me (I am sure that's why they're sliced in sandwich portions anyway). I've seen folks spread mayonnaise on bread, multiple slices of ham and cheese, mustard, ketchup, more mayo and one more slice of bread to keep it all together. It makes my stomach turn I tell you.

I have mentioned footlong subs® (which leave the Big Mac® a pity middleweight) in the Footlong chapter.

A couple of modest sandwiches are ideal for breakfast or lunch. I would advise school cafeterias to serve sandwich buffets for lunch instead of Domino's®, Pizza Hut®, McDonald's®, Subway® or Taco Bell®. Just imagine, serving kids Fast Food for lunch, how dare you!

See also Footlong.

Sauce

Sauce comes from the Latin word salsus, which means salted! It adds to the flavor and "looks" of a dish. There are a ton of different sauces but most of them have one thing in common; high carbs, sodium, and/or fat content. Using sauce is not really a problem if you can keep it to the recommended serving size.

Product	Serving Size	Calories	Fat	Carbs.	Sodium
Apple sauce	1/2 cup (128 g)	110	0 g	27 g	19 mg
RDI			6%	0%	9%	1%
BBQ sauce	1 packet (9.3 g)	14	0 g	3.4 g	104 mg
RDI			1%	0%	1%	4%
Gravy, white	1/2 cup (125 g)	184	13.3 g	11.5 g	443 mg
RDI			9%	20%	4%	18%
Hollandaise sauce	1 tbsp (14.8ml - 0.5 oz)	94	10 g	1 g	64 mg
RDI			5%	15%	0%	3%
Hot sauce	1 tsp (4.9ml - 0.17 oz)	0	0 g	0 g	124 mg
RDI			0%	0%	0%	5%
Soy sauce	1 packet (8.9 g)	5	0 g	0.9 g	502mg
RDI			0%	0%	0%	21%
Spaghetti sauce	1 serving (125 g - 1/2 cup)	109	3.4 g	17.2 g	513 mg
RDI			5%	5%	6%	21%

Source:

http://caloriecount.about.com

http://en.wikipedia.org/wiki/Sauce
http://www.livestrong.com

Sausage

The worldwide custom of preserving meat, and especially animal parts we don't want to eat consciously. Usually high fat and salt content and low nutritional value. Popular already among the ancient Greeks and Romans, Epicharmus wrote a comedy about it 500 B.C. called "The Orya" (the sausage).

A popular old-time winter recipe from The Netherlands is Boerenkool (borecole/kale) and potato mash with Rookworst (smoked sausage), the kale is harvested right after the first frosty night.

There are tons of different sausagesthe British "Black Pudding" (a blood sausage), the German "Bratwurst" (there's even a Bratwurst museum) or what about the Scottish "Haggis"?

Though sausage consumption is enormous all around the world, the cooked (fatty) breakfast sausage or patty seems to be restricted to English-speaking and Eastern-European countries as far as I can tell.

Nutritional data on various sausages from random manufacturers:

Product	Serving Size	Calories	Fat	Carbs.	Sodium
Johnsonville®					
Bratwurst, Original	1 link (85g - 3oz)	270	22 g	2 g	810 mg
RDI		14%	34%	1%	34%
Omaha Steaks®					
Breakfast sausage link	1 link (48g - 1.7oz)	210	21 g	1 g	400 mg
RDI		11%	32%	0%	17%
Jimmy Dean®					
Breakfast sausage patty	1 patty (35g - 1.2oz)	120	12 g	0.5 g	305 mg
RDI		6%	18%	0%	13%
Syracuse®					
Italian sausage, sweet	1 link (114g - 4oz)	280	22 g	2 g	660 mg
RDI		14%	34%	1%	28%
Hillshire Farm®					
Polish kielbasa sausage	1 link (76g - 2.7oz)	250	22g	4 g	670 mg
RDI		13%	34%	1%	28%
Bob Evans®					
Turkey sausage link	1 link (45g - 1.6oz)	72	4 g	1 g	404 mg
RDI		4%	6%	0%	17%

Source:

http://www2.bobevans.com/website%5Cnutritionals.nsf/Websearch?SearchView&Qu

ery=sausage&SearchOrder=1 http://caloriecount.about.com
http://en.wikipedia.org/wiki/Black_pudding
http://en.wikipedia.org/wiki/Epicharmus_of_Kos

http://en.wikipedia.org/wiki/Orya
http://en.wikipedia.org/wiki/Sausage
http://foodmood.over-blog.net/article-american-sausages-53913640.html

http://www.gomeat.com/products http://jimmydean.com/products/Sausage
http://www.johnsonville.com/products/original-bratwurst.html
http://www.livestrong.com/thedailyplate
http://www.livestrong.com/thedailyplate/nutrition-calories/food/syracuses-sausage-
company/sweet-italian-sausage-links
http://www.omahasteaks.com/gifs/NutritionAnalysis.pdf
http://penelope.uchicago.edu/Thayer/E/Roman/Texts/Athenaeus/3C.html*

Smoothies

See Soft Drinks

Snacks

Researchers at the University of North Carolina discovered that on average more than 27 percent (!) of American children's daily calories are coming from snacks! Half of the kids snack 4 or more times a day. Sixty percent of Americans eat snack food regularly, getting about 20 percent of their calories from snacks. Europeans consume about 10% less snacks than Americans.

Trivial fact: the word "snack" comes from the Dutch word "snak", is means something like "to yearn".

Here's a compilation of some favorite snacks:

Product	Serving Size	Calories	Fat	Carbs.	Sodium
Mars® almond candy bar,	1 bar (50g, 1.76oz)	234	11.5 g	31.4 g	85 mg
RDI		11%	18%	10%	4%
Oreo® Cookies	1 cookie (34 g)	160	7 g	24 g	180 mg
RDI		8%	11%	8%	8%
Jelly beans®	10 beans (11 g)	41	0 g	10.3 g	6 mg
RDI		2%	0%	3%	0%
M&M® chocolate	1 packet (48 g - 1.69 oz)	236	10.1 g	34.2 g	29 mg
RDI		12%	16%	11%	1%
Peanuts, salted	1 cup (144 g)	863	75.6 g	22 g	461 mg
RDI		43%	**116%**	7%	19%
Popcorn, oil popped	1 cup (11 g)	64	4.8 g	5 g	116 mg
RDI		3%	7%	2%	6%
Potato chips	12 chips (28 g - 1 oz)	150	10 g	15 g	180 mg
RDI		8%	15%	5%	8%
Rold Gold® pretzels	17 pretzels (28 g - 1 oz)	115	1 g	23.5 g	450 mg
RDI		6%	2%	8%	19%

Where is the fruit you might ask? Well so did I!

Also see Candybars, Chocolate, Ice-cream, Potato-chips

Source:
http://en.wikipedia.org/wiki/List_of_snack_foods

http://en.wikipedia.org/wiki/Snack_food http://www.faqs.org/nutrition/Diab-Em/Dietary-Trends-American.html

http://findarticles.com/p/articles/mi_m0EIN/is_2006_Sept_4/ai_n16703092/
http://www.healthnews.com/family-health/child-health/us-kids-increasing-daily-snack-consumption-4123.html
http://www.lifeintheusa.com/food/snackfoods.htm

Soda-pop / Soft drinks

A non-alcoholic beverage containing water and flavoring, often carbonated and sweetened.

1942, U.S. annual production of carbonated soft drinks was about 60 12-ounce (355 ml) servings per person; in 2004 production had risen to 557 12-ounce servings per person!

USDA has recommended that, depending on their calorie intake, people consume no more than 6 to 10 percent of their calories from added sugars. For example, people who consume 2,000 calories per day should limit themselves to 10 teaspoons (40g, 1.41 oz) of added sugars. That's about what's in one average soft drink: A 12-ounce Coke or Pepsi has 40 grams of sugar, while Mountain Dew has 46 grams and Sunkist Orange Soda has 52 grams.

Fruit Drinks

You might not expect it, but most fruit drinks, including the "no added sugar" versions, contain just as much, if not more sugar than carbonated soft drinks. Isn't that a surprise? Some researchers call it "Liquid Candy". As I mentioned before, 100% juice contains the same amount of sugar as Coke or even more. Check the nutrition labels on your "health product".

Product	Serving Size	Calories	Carbs.	Carbs. from sugar	Sugar (teaspoons)
Cola	12 oz (355 ml)	145	40 g (139%)	40 g	10
Orange Juice	12 oz (355 ml)	165	39 g (139%)	33 g	8
Apple Juice	12 oz (355 ml)	165	42 g (174%)	39 g	10
Cherry Juice	12 oz (355 ml)	210	49.5 g (176%)	37.5 g	9
Grape Juice	12 oz (355 ml)	240	60 g (200%)	58.5 g	1

Percentages R.D.I. according to the F.D.A.

Source: hookedonjuice.com

Smoothies

Everything your hear or read about smoothies makes one think this is by far one of the healthiest drinks; Fresh fruit or veggies, natural ingredients and lots of vitamins. This might be true for some of the more sensible smoothies, especially the unsweetened ones. But be aware...

Calories! Check the labels folks. One McDonalds® small banana/strawberry smoothie has about the same amount of calories as a medium Coke.

The Smoothie King® small "Stay Healthy" choices (20oz) are good for at least a 25% of your daily calories, carbs and sugar needs. Do you call that "Stay Healthy"?

Smoothies can be a tasty and healthy part of your diet, if you get them from the right places, or if you make them yourself.

Yogurt Drinks

One of the fastest growing food and beverage products worldwide.

So-called "probiotic" products like Activia® and Yakult® carry, besides the Lactobacillus casei (Immunitas for Americans) bacteria, a troubling 17 grams of sugar per 3.3 fl oz (100 ml) or more. The "25% Less Sugar Lowfat" versions still contain as much sugar as the same amount of coke. Yakult bottles in the USA are 23% larger than in Europe.

Health benefits of these products are still debated.

Also see Cola, Sugar and Syrup

Source:
http://www.consumerreports.org/cro/food/food-shopping/dairy/kids-yogurts-with-less-sugar/overview/kids-yogurts-with-less-sugar-ov.htm
http://dannon.com/ourproducts.aspx
http://en.wikipedia.org/wiki/Actimel
http://en.wikipedia.org/wiki/Smoothie
http://en.wikipedia.org/wiki/Yakult
http://en.wikipedia.org/wiki/Yoghurt
http://www.fruitjuicefacts.org/
http://www.hookedonjuice.com/
http://www.nutraingredients-usa.com/Consumer-Trends/Yogurt-drinks-are-leading-food-and-beverage-product-ACNielsen
http://www.probiotics-lovethatbug.com/danactive.html
http://www.smoothieking.com/downloads/Nutritional_Guide_2010.pdf
http://www.thatsfit.com/2010/07/14/mcdonalds-smoothies-more-calories-than-a-cheeseburger/

Steak

American steak sizes are totally out of proportion nowadays. (Not because I'm European, they really are!) The U.S. Department of Agriculture recommends a standard steak serving size of 3 oz (85g)! Restaurants serve steaks from 8 oz (227 g) up to a staggering 18 oz (510 g) steaks! The American Institute on Cancer Research recommends eating less than 18 oz of red meat per week.

There are many crazy "steak challenges" where you eat inhuman amounts of meat usually in a fixed amount of time. To name a couple:

72 oz "World Famous Big Texan" (4.5 lbs, 2,041 g), 5,400 cal Sirloin The Big Texan Steak Ranch - Amarillo, Texas

96 oz "Texas Cattle Company 6 lbs Challenge" (2,721 g), 7,200 cal Sirloin Texas Cattle Company - Lakeland, Florida

120 oz "The World's Largest Steak" (7.5 lbs, 3,402 g), 9,000 cal Ribeye Gregory's Steakhouse - Allentown, Pennsylvania Officially a 4 person steak but according to the USDA should serve 40 people (at 3 oz each)

There are even, in my opinion ridiculous, TV-shows, where someone takes up a lot of these crazy food-challenges and contests, and seems to be very proud of it. A glorification of obesity! Again, please don't subject your body to these very, very unhealthy and insane eating contests!

Source:
http://www.aicr.org/site/PageServer?pagename=elements_red_processed_meat
http://www.bigtexan.com/free72.html
http://www.cnpp.usda.gov/Publications/DietaryGuidelines/2000/2000DGBrochure
HowMuch.pdf http://en.wikipedia.org/wiki/T-bone_steak
http://www.gregoryssteakhouse.com/monstersteaks.html
http://www.livestrong.com/article/299625-t-bone-steak-nutrition/
http://www.steak-enthusiast.com/2010/02/6-belt-busting-steak-challenges/
http://www.talkofthetownrestaurants.com/texas_lakeland.html

Super-size

Watch the 2004 Academy Award-nominated movie "Super Size Me" by Morgan Spurlock if you haven't already.

See also XL.

Syrup

Syrup is basically water with dissolved sugar, heated so more sugar then actually possible can be used. Usually named after the plant that provided the sugar i.e. corn syrup or maple syrup.

Aunt Jemima® Syrup, Regular, serving size 2 tbsp (30g, 1oz) holds 110 cal, 30mg sodium (1%) and 27g carbs (9%)Ihop® Pancake Syrup, serving size 4 tbsp (60g, 2oz) holds 230 cal, 230mg sodium (10%) and 58g carbs (18%)Ruby's Diner® Pancake Syrup, serving size small pitcher (2 1/2 fl oz, 100g) holds 287 cal, 83mg sodium (3%) and 76g carbs (25%)

Percentages R.D.I. according to the F.D.A.

High Fructose Corn Syrup - H.F.C.S.

In the USA, since the 1980's, high-fructose corn syrup has replaced sugar in many foods (from bread and soft drinks to ketchup and what not), mainly because it is cheaper as a result of a combination of corn subsidies and sugar tariffs and quotas. It is virtually impossible to avoid consuming HFCS nowadays. This trend is not seen in other parts of the world. The average American consumed 1/2 pound of high fructose corn syrup in 1970. By the mid-1990s, that figure has jumped to 55.3 pounds of HFCS per person (USDA).

"America's sweet tooth increased 39 percent between 1950-59 and 2000 as use of corn sweeteners octupled."(1)

There's a health controversy about the usage of HFCS. When ingested, unlike other carbohydrates, it travels straight to the liver, which turns the fructose straight into stored fat, skipping the pancreas insulin production (which controls our blood sugar level). Meaning: we keep on eating food that is converted into fat but our brain does not receive the signals that we're full. In other words: It's cheap and fattening!

Again I plead for responsible food production where quality should be more important than finding ever-cheaper ingredients. Consumers" health should be more important than stockholders" bank accounts!

Source:
1. http://www.usda.gov/factbook/chapter2.pdf

http://caloriecount.about.com
http://www.dulu.info/gezondheid/2010/09/Is-High-Fructose-Corn-Syrup-Slecht-voor-Mij.html
http://en.wikipedia.org/wiki/High-fructose_corn_syrup
http://en.wikipedia.org/wiki/Syrup
http://healthmad.com/nutrition/dangers-of-high-fructose-corn-syrup/
http://www.livestrong.com/thedailyplate
http://www.menshealth.com
http://www.wikihow.com/Avoid-High-Fructose-Corn-Syrup

T.

Take-out

Americans eat out, on average, about 209 times per year. This includes dining in restaurants and getting take-out. Take-out is usually fast food, often in much bigger portions than necessary. "One size fits all". Seven out of ten restaurants use the cheap and highly saturated corn oil for cooking. Lots of sugars, fat, starch and water (pasta sauce) are used as extra ingredients to increase volumes. Commercial business seems to be more interested in selling cheap fulfilling meals rather than healthy ones.

Every time people tell me about food places, I hear: "The food is really good there", "they've got great food", and so on. Nobody tells you the food tastes good or great, which is actually what is meant here.

The term "good food" is a "homonym"; it wrongfully leads you to think that the food is actually good for you. It makes you believe you're eating something healthy and nutritious when you probably aren't. "Really good ribs" for instance is a contradiction in terms

See also Junk food.

Source:
http://en.wikipedia.org/wiki/Take-out http://www.ehow.com/facts_5894661_corn-oil-unhealthy_.html
https://stores.healthmart.com/oakleypharmacy/RelatedItems/6,635088
http://www.wisegeek.com/how-do-steaks-served-in-restaurants-compare-with-recommended-portion-sizes.htm

TV Dinners

Food for the lazy singles! Pop one in the microwave and a couple of minutes later you're eating a "meal" in front of your TV or computer. Home-cooking in the 21st Century. There's "no time to cook" nowadays is the pity excuse for eating these abominations. How can you not have time to prepare your own meals? What can be more important than taking care of yourself? (Food for thought I hope)

The TV dinner developed in 1953 for C.A. Swanson & Sons® grew to a generic trademark worldwide. The package featured an image of a TV set and folks would often eat them while watching TV. There are tons of frozen dinners now, some healthier than others, some contain less than one tablespoon of vegetables.

Freezing food lowers the taste; this is usually compensated by extra salt and fat. Low calorie dinners can easily fool you because they can leave you unsatisfied and ready for more. Choose wisely if you feel the need to include microwave-meals in your diet.

Product	Serving Size	Calories	Fat	Carbs.	Cholestorol	Sodium
Hungry Man - Swanson®						
Boneless White Meat						
Fried Chicken Dinner	1 dinner	710	29 g	86 g	165 mg	2160 mg
RDI		36%	45%	29%	55%	90%
Michelina's Lean Gourmet®	1 dinner					
Cheese Stuffed Rigatoni	227 g	220	6 g	33 g	30 mg	510 mg
RDI		11%	9%	11%	10%	21%
Marie Callender's®	1 dinner					
Country Fried Chicken & Gravy	454 g	560	26 g	61 g	60 mg	1590 mg
RDI		28%	40%	20%	20%	66%
Boston Market®						
Meatloaf with Homestyle	1 dinner					
Mashed Potatoes & Gravy	453 g	710	42 g	53 g	95 mg	1590 mg
RDI		36%	64%	18%	31%	66%
Banquet®	1 dinner					
Salisbury Steak Dinner	269.3 g	290	16 g	25 g	30 mg	1100 mg
RDI		15%	25%	8%	10%	46%
Stouffers®	1 dinner					
White Meat Chicken Pot Pie	283 g	630	35 g	57 g	55 mg	1020 mg
RDI		32%	54%	19%	19%	43%

At the present time, Michelina's® and Swanson® have no nutritional data published on their websites!

Source:
http://www.associatedcontent.com/topic/64613/frozen_dinner.html?cat=51
http://www.bostonmarketfrozen.com/Product-View.aspx?ID=1
http://caloriecount.about.com/calories-swanson-hungry-man-dinner-boneless-i115928
http://www.conagrafoods.com/consumer/brands/getBrand.do?page=banquet
http://www.copperwiki.org/index.php/TV_Dinners
http://en.wikipedia.org/wiki/TV_dinner

http://findarticles.com/p/articles/mi_m0813/is_5_32/ai_n13806479/
http://www.livestrong.com/thedailyplate/nutrition-calories/food/marie-callenders/country-fried-chicken-and-gravy/
http://www.livestrong.com/thedailyplate/nutrition-calories/food/swanson/hungry-man-boneless-white-meat-fried-chicken-dinner/
http://www.michelinas.com/ProductByBrand_LG_10626_Cheese_Stuffed_Rigatoni_1Lean_Gourmet.aspx http://nutritionknowhow.org/wordpress/?p=1582
http://www.redandblack.com/news/light-frozen-meals-not-instant-healthy-choice
http://www.stouffers.com/products/nutrition/186/White-Meat-Chicken-Pot-Pie.aspx
http://www.toaster.net/~jule/tvdinner.html

U.

Ultra-Thin Slices (and lots of them)

"The thinner the slice, the higher the price!" - An elderly woman's wise remark. Ultra-thin sliced luncheon meat does not contribute to lower calorie and fat intake simply because you are going to use more of them. The enormous amount of deli-meat and cheese you Americans put on your sandwiches is unbelievable anyway.

Also see Sandwiches.

USA vs EUROPE

No competition!!

The following table is a comparison of some American and European health and eating habits that struck me as notable.

	U.S.A.	EUROPE
Average Daily Calorie Intake	3770	3263
Average Daily Fat Intake	5.8oz (164g)	4.7oz (132g)
Average Daily Protein Intake	4.1oz (116g)	3.6oz (103g)
Average Small Soda Serving	16oz (0.47 ltr)	8.5oz (0.25 ltr)
Average Steak Portion Size	8oz (227g)	5oz (150g)
Obesity - Adults	34%	17%
Overweight (incl. obese) - Total	64%	48%
Daily trips on foot or bicycle	9.4%	33%

Source:
http://www.cdc.gov/nchs/fastats/overwt.htm
http://www.cdc.gov/nchs/data/hestat/obesity_child_07_08/obesity_child_07_08.pdf
http://en.wikipedia.org/wiki/Obesity_in_the_United_States
http://www.ers.usda.gov/data-products/chart-
gallery/detail.aspx?chartId=36272&ref=collection#.Ut92Bvbb8y4
http://www.fao.org/economic/ess/publications-studies/statistical-yearbook/en/
http://www.kvsmith.com/1/2008/01/why-americans-a.html
http://www.iotf.org/database/documents/v2PDFforwebsiteEU27.pdf

http://today.msnbc.msn.com/id/38959769/ns/today-today_health/
http://www.northjersey.com/news/health/102603249_New_Jersey_could_help_solve
_obesity_by_making_it_easier_for_people_to_walk_or_bike.html
http://www.reuters.com/article/idUSN0131635120071002

V.

Vanilla

Ok, I'm busted, there's hardly any food with a "v" except for vanilla and it is not very fattening by itself.

Did you know that most vanilla products contain hardly any real vanilla nowadays? Up to 95% of the "vanilla" products actually contain artificial vanillin, produced from lignin, a constituent of wood, which is a byproduct of the paper industry. Think about it the next time you're enjoying your vanilla ice-cream.

Source:

http://en.wikipedia.org/wiki/Lignin
http://en.wikipedia.org/wiki/Vanilla

http://en.wikipedia.org/wiki/Vanillin
http://www.vanilla.com

W.

Waffles

Belgian Waffles, what a treat! And that's what it is; it's not a meal. Not even with bacon and eggs! You wouldn't order apple pie for breakfast/dinner would you?

And again the portion sizes...

A circular waffle iron divides the waffle visually into different portions. American waffle houses seem to overlook the fact that these are the actual serving size portions, instead they'll serve you four waffles still connected as one huge waffle! You won't find them like that anywhere in Belgium.

Product	Serving Size	Cal.	Fat	Sat. Fat	Carbs.	Chol.	Sodium	Protein
IHOP® Belgian Waffle	1 Waffle	390	19 g	15 g	48 mg	140 mg	820 mg	8 g
RDI		200%	200%	600%	160%	740%	350%	160%
Denny's® Belgian Waffle	1 platter	650	50 g	24 g	31 mg	282 mg	1130 mg	20 g
RDI		330%	110%	150%	100%	650%	500%	400%
Waffle House® Belgian Waffle	1 Waffle	314	15 g	3 g	45 mg	3 mg	3 mg	5.9 g
RDI		160%	160%	30%	120%	30%	30%	120%

Nutritional data above is without butter, syrup or fruit topping.

Waffle House ® does not publish nutritional data on their website! Makes you wonder doesn't it?

Source:
http://caloriecount.about.com
http://www.dennys.com/LiveImages/enProductImage_900.pdf
http://en.wikipedia.org/wiki/Waffle
http://www.livestrong.com/thedailyplate/nutrition-calories/food/ihop/belgian-waffle/
http://www.livestrong.com/thedailyplate/nutrition-calories/food/waffle-house/waffle/

Whipped cream

Perfect topping for a coffee, cake, ice cream or most desserts, and to spoil yourself! It's made by whipping cream (with 30% fat or over) so tiny air bubbles can be caught between the fat droplets. (Does that sound as gross to you as it does to me?)

One tbsp of heavy whipping cream with 36% milk fat contains over 50cal and the 40% version has 60cal and 17% R.D.I. of saturated fat. This is the recommended serving size.

Skip the cream on your coffee next time and save a good 120cal.

Source:

http://en.wikipedia.org/wiki/Lignin

http://en.wikipedia.org/wiki/Vanilla http://en.wikipedia.org/wiki/Vanillin
http://www.livestrong.com/article/257399-heavy-whipping-cream-nutrition/
http://www.livestrong.com/article/71048-drink-coffee-healthy-way/
http://www.vanilla.com

X.

XXL

XL in food means XXL in size.

Male: A regular? I'm not regular, I'm a MAN, a real man, I can afford it, YEAH give me a BIG/LARGE/JUMBO/GIANT/XL/XXL/XXXL/MAN-SIZE/KING-SIZE/SUPERSIZED, hell why not a MAMMOTH SIZE EXTRAVAGANZA!

Female: Well just maybe one more. I know I shouldn't but it's so CREAMY, DELICIOUS, FULL FLAVORED, HEAVENLY, JUICY, RICH, SWEET, TASTY, hmmm almost SEXUAL PLEASURE!

BIGGER does NOT necessarily mean BETTER!!! It seldom does in reference to food...

Giant, enormous portions sizes are not cool! They are pathetic. Over the top portions might impress a five year old into thinking they are something great, but if you are a grown-up and still think that 64oz cokes or double half pounder cheeseburgers are way cool, you're missing the point and need some serious growing up to do. Eating more that any person in their right mind knows is good for them is not cool, it's stupid.

Source:

http://en.wikipedia.org/wiki/Sugar
http://www.usda.gov/factbook/chapter2.pdf

Y.

Yams

Sweet potatos (Convolvulaceae) are often referred to as yams (Dioscoreaceae) in the US, they are not the same thing though.

Cooked yams contain a little over 1 cal per gram (0.035oz), sweet potatos little less than 1 cal/g. One average yam should be around 1oz (283g).

Source:
http://en.wikipedia.org/wiki/Sweet_potato
http://en.wikipedia.org/wiki/Yam_(vegetable)
http://caloriecount.about.com/calories-yam-i11601
http://www.livestrong.com/thedailyplate/search/?q=sweet+potato&mode=tdp
http://www.livestrong.com/thedailyplate/nutrition-calories/food/generic/yam-cooked-no-salt-added/

Yogurt Drinks

See Soft Drinks

You

You are of course the most important factor in taking care of yourself. And excuse me for saying this but you are lazy! We are all lazy. Times have changed a lot since we don't have to spend much physical energy to hunt and gather our food anymore. We sit behind computers and TV screens with remote controls; we order our food lying on the couch and complain if we have to wait half an hour for someone to bring it right to our front doors. We buy factory-packed "fresh" sandwiches, fruits, veggies and drinks. We drive our cars constantly, using drive-thru banking and fast-food places so we won't even have to get out. We'd rather eat cheap and a lot than healthy and nutritious, and we accept that companies produce low quality food this way. We watch more sports than we participate in. We are growing bigger and fatter every day and we're wondering why?

You can change all of this! Yes You!

You can start eating and living more consciously! You can make sure that you AND your kids have enough exercise. You can start eating more local products so your fruits won't have to sail halfway across the world. You can start demanding higher nutritional quality food and regular size portions from producers. You can require your government to change food laws to benefit people's health instead of taking lobbyists money.

Finally, you can reassess your high demands; eat some frozen fish so markets won't have to throw away 75% of the "fresh fish" because you don't buy it. Or buy a pear with a little spot on it and cut it out before you eat it, instead of having the store throw it away because it wasn't perfect enough for you. (I know... I am straying from the subject but it is food for thought for sure)

Z.

Zero-sugar

No sugar intake at all is not possible. We all need sugars, fats and calories to live. There's no need to take it to the extreme and jump to the other side of the scale.

Most artificial sweeteners are debated as potentially dangerous to our health. There are a number of different sweeteners available today, not all of them artificial. In the US, six intensely-sweet sugar substitutes have been F.D.A. approved for use:

Artificial: Acesulfame Potassium (K) (e.g., Sunett®, Sweet One®) Aspartame (e.g., Equal®, NutraSweet®) Neotame (e.g., NutraSweet®) Saccharin (e.g., Sweet'N Low®) Sucralose (e.g., Splenda®, Altern®)

Herbal: Stevia (e.g., Only Sweet®, PureVia®, Rebiana®, and Truvia®)

Maltitol and Sorbitol are commonly found in toothpaste and mouth wash.

In other countries, Xylitol, Cyclamate and Stevia are widely used.

I won't go into the potential dangers of using artificial sweeteners but personally I would rather be safe than sorry. The fact is that people consume too much sugary products. And instead of cutting down on consumption, we would rather change a product so we can still overindulge.

Also see Diet-soda, Low-Sugar and Sugar.

Source:

http://en.wikipedia.org/wiki/Sugar_substitute

http://www.mcdonaldsmenu.info
http://naturalbias.com/are-you-being-fooled-by-zero-calorie-sodas/
http://www.nature.com/oby/journal/v16/n8/abs/oby2008284a.html
http://www.sweetpoison.com/aspartame-sweeteners.html

Conclusion

Portion sizes, portion sizes, portion sizes! The American "*one size fits all*" portions seem to be fit for the biggest Americans people, not the average person! You can eat anything you want, really, if you eat moderately. Take another look at your personal diet, calculate your personal nutritional needs and do not overeat. Maybe try to find other menu's, dishes, meals, foods, that might be "un-American" and non-commercial but will be much better for your health.

If you have any comments, remarks, or tips, ideas, please feel free to let me know: abc@hermanbrockjr.com

ABOUT THE AUTHOR

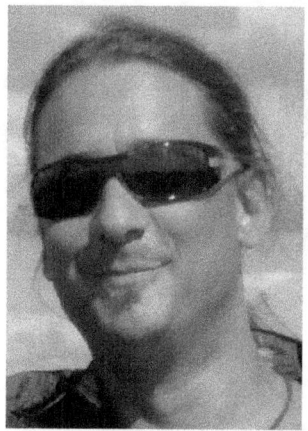

Herman de Brock jr. was born September 18th 1970 in Winterswijk and grew up in Terneuzen, The Netherlands. His career as a musician and guitar teacher allowed him to make frequent visits and small tours to the USA, where he found that maintaining a "normal diet" according to European standards was quite difficult. A spontaneous pneumothorax (collapsed lung) forced Herman to quit smoking, resulting in a craving for fattening foods which caused him to gain over 70 lbs in one year. After working hard to reduce this excess weight he felt the need to tell the world, and especially America, how fattening and high-caloric even the most common foods actually are, resulting in The "*ABC of Obesity*". Written in English; the author's second language.